COLOUR HEALING MANUAL

PAULINE WILLS

COLOUR HEALING MANUAL

THE COMPLETE COLOUR THERAPY
TEACHING PROGRAMME

PIATKUS

Photo credits – *Plate 1*: courtesy of Alfred Pasieka/Science Photo Library; *Plates 2–4*: Rodney Paull

First published in 2000 by
Judy Piatkus (Publishers) Ltd
5 Windmill Street, London W1P 1HF
E-mail: info@piatkus.co.uk

For the latest news and information on all our titles
visit our new website at www.piatkus.co.uk

A catalogue record for this book is available from the British Library

ISBN 0-7499-1963-9

Designed by Paul Saunders
Illustrations by Rodney Paull
Typeset by Wyvern 21 Ltd, Bristol
Printed and bound in Great Britain by
The Bath Press, Bath, Somerset

To Lily Cornford

CONTENTS

INTRODUCTION

COLOUR IS A PHENOMENON that is with us every second of our life. During our waking hours nature surrounds us with the vast range of colours which she displays in flowers, trees, rocks, minerals, the variegated plumage of birds and the multi-coloured designs exhibited throughout the animal and reptile kingdom. In our homes we mimic these colours with dyes in upholstery and furnishings and in the clothes we wear. At night when we sleep, colour appears in our dreams and during the 24 hours of each day, our own electromagnetic field, the aura, cloaks us with an array of ever-changing colours, responsible at one level for feeding the systems of the physical body with pranic energy.

I like to think of colour as a large tree. The darkness from the earth travels up the tree's roots to meet the light of day. Here the darkness and light interact to produce the spectral colours for the tree's trunk. Each colour then splits into its many shades to form the branches. The shades of red found at the heat end of the visible spectrum form the lowest branches and the shades of violet the upper ones. The colours which lie between these two colours shape the branches in between. This tree can now be metaphorically linked to a human being or to the different paths associated with colour and light.

We can also liken the tree's branches to the many levels of colour consciousness that exist in today's population. Becoming aware that other aspects and levels exist motivates us to explore further in order to expand our awareness and heighten our sensitivity. Having said this, I feel that it is important for you to know that the level and aspect of colour that you are personally working with is right for you at this present time.

If we use our tree in this aspect, the lower branches represent those of you who work with or understand colour at a physical level. This encompasses scientists whose aim is to understand the physics of light and colour, the effect these have on the atomic structure of the human, animal and plant kingdom, also those of you who use colour creatively to enhance your home, garden or for personal beautification through fashion and make up.

Climbing to the next layer of branches we find those who have heightened their sensitivity to colour and are conscious of how each colour affects them physically, mentally and emotionally. These are the people who are aware at all times of the colours they need to keep them healthy and in a state of balance. Some of the ways they utilise these colours are with visualisation, meditation, colour breathing and through the colours of the clothes they wear. The colours that we wear take on a completely different meaning at this level of our understanding. They are not worn to enhance our skin tone or hair colouring but as a filter for the absorption of the needed colour through the pores of the skin. Indeed, the colour worn is frequently a colour that the wearer does not particularly like – but not liking a colour does not mean that we don't need it for our well-being.

At the top of the tree we find those who have realised and experienced the spiritual aspects of colour. These people are awake to the knowledge that they are beings of light and therefore need light for their well-being. Frequently they are able to see the interplay of auric colours surrounding their fellow human beings, animals and plants, and with this gift are able to ascertain the colours an individual is lacking and therefore needs. One of the questions that I am frequently asked by students is whether they must be able to see the aura before embarking upon a colour practitioner's course. The answer to this question is no. Part of the course is designed to help students heighten their colour sensitivity and to appreciate and understand colour at all of its many levels. Those who embark upon a colour therapy course prematurely will fail to complete it, and this is right for them. Perhaps at a later stage in their life they will continue with the course or they may choose a different path, but one which embraces the knowledge and understanding gained through the part of the training they undertook.

One of my students enrolled for the colour practitioner course because she wished to know more about colour and its therapeutic properties. She was a very intelligent lady working with one of the sciences. She was sceptical about the healing power of colour and stated at the beginning of the course that she did not wish to qualify as a colour practitioner but wished to learn more about colour. Halfway through the course she was treated with and treated other students with colour. She admitted that this experience made her conscious of the powerful effect that colour had on her and those she was working with. Part way through her second year of training she left the course because she had discovered another way of using colour which she resonated to. In her letter she thanked us for helping her to realise the power and potential of colour and said that without the knowledge and experience gained from the course she would not have discovered the path that now felt right for her.

If we now liken the tree to ourselves, the dense spectrum of colours forming the trunk are the colours penetrating our dense physical body which is earthed to this planet by our own roots. The lower branches displaying the paler shades of red represent the etheric sheath, the blueprint for the physical body. The ones above these, that are tinted with the paler shades of orange, portray the feelings which fill our emotional body; then come those vibrating to the subtle shades of yellow and green, standing for the constant stream of thoughts constituting our mental body, and the narrow branches at the top of the tree, displaying the ethereal colours of indigo and violet, form our spiritual aspect. For the tree to be healthy and strong its colours need to be made clear and luminous from both the nourishment it receives from the earth and the energy from the sun. The same applies to us but we also need to integrate the earth energy with the energy of our spiritual sun to create a greater sense of wholeness.

If we compare the branches of the tree to the many facets of colour and the facets to colour's many paths, then we begin to understand that each path is but a small portion of the whole, a portion which needs to be acknowledged and respected for the part it plays. Each path has its own unique way of working with and teaching colour and will attract those who are ready to hear what it has to say. As individuals grow and develop, they will move on to a path with teaching in greater depth or to one which explores another facet. This might be the use of colour in design, in art, with sound, in heraldry, in minerals or in fashion, to name but a few. Exploring other aspects of colour does not necessarily involve working exclusively with these, but the knowledge gleaned enhances that which is already known.

Occasionally branches on a tree wither and die through playing host to another plant or because of invasion by insects. In the world of colour this process can be compared to the use of colour power for manipulative purposes, where colour is used to entice the public to buy simply to increase productivity.

In advertising and packaging colour is used to arrest the attention and make an impact on the mind. A common choice for cigarette packets is red, to give smokers the feeling that a cigarette will make them feel more lively by increasing their energy. Nearly all financial institutions use dark blue in their advertising, a colour which appeals to an innate need for security and therefore puts over to the client the notion of the companies' trustworthiness. In advertising black and gold are used a great deal because black represents the ultimate in sophistication and gold is thought to be the highest colour. Max Luscher, Professor of Psychology at the University of Basle, regards black as the colour representing the ultimate surrender or relinquishment.

In the food industry, taste is linked in a big way to colour, making it an important factor in marketing. The skins of both lemons and oranges are coloured to make them more appealing. The normal colour of canned processed peas is greyish green, but to make them appear more nutritious and tasty green colouring is added. The colour red is associated with high flavour and in some countries tomatoes and other red vegetables are grown commercially in brightly coloured varieties and even though the process by which they are grown renders them tasteless, their colour sells them. Over many years a clear blue on white has been used for packaging dairy produce. These colours suggest coolness and hygiene, but the use of the wrong shade of blue or green would bring mould and decay to mind, making the product a non-starter.

The colours which exert a measurable effect on the autonomic nervous system, stimulating the appetite, are red, orange, yellow and brown. This renders these colours a favourite for marketing and selling food. Another colour which is thought to be very appetising is a golden brown and because of this the baking and roasting of bread, nuts and cereals is precisely controlled so that the finished item is neither too light nor too dark. If marketers wish to promote their cereal as giving the body warmth on a cold winter's day, they package it in orange and red, but for a sunshine, energising cereal, yellow is used.

Becoming aware of how we are being manipulated by the food industry and marketing boards through the medium of colour should make us stop and ask ourselves what nutritional value is in the food we are buying and whether we are buying it for this or because it looks appetising. The number of people who are turning to organically produced food suggests that the population is starting to awaken to the fact that they are being manipulated into buying devitalised, chemically produced and coloured food which is reaping untold wealth for the food industry.

My own introduction into the world of colour was through yoga. I had been unwell for some time and turned to yoga in desperation as I was tired of taking drugs and getting nowhere with conventional medicine. At this time yoga was not as popular as it is today, but I was very fortunate in finding an Indian teacher who had spent most of his life studying and practising the many aspects of the subject. Through regular practice of the postures, coupled with the breathing techniques linked with these postures and work on the relevant chakras through the colours which radiated from them, I slowly recovered. Through my study of yoga I came to realise that the asanas or postures which are taught in hatha yoga work with clearing and opening the chakras or energy centres and strengthen the physical body for the greater flow of energy these postures generate. Each of the seven chakras radiates one of the spectral colours, and using colour visualisations and breathing techniques with the postures amplified their effect. Through this I began to realise the power of colour and I started to use it in other aspects of my life. The results I experienced fascinated me and I thirsted for more knowledge and a greater understanding of the vibrational energies of colour and ways in which these could be used to further help myself and others.

By chance, if anything ever happens this way, I was informed by a friend of a colour course that was being run quite close to where I was then living. When I telephoned for details, I discovered that it was being held at the Maitreya School of Colour Healing, which was run by Lily Cornford together with Ronald Leech, known to us all as Joseph. I enrolled for the course and throughout its duration learnt a great deal from Lily, a very astute and gifted lady. Attending these lectures became the highlight of my week. After qualifying to practise colour therapy, along with the other newly qualified practitioners, I worked for the first year at the Maitreya School alongside Lily. It was a very enlightening experience and one I thank her for. During the time that I worked there the very young through to the old were treated for a vast range of ailments and my experience and my knowledge grew. Lily always showed a wonderful sense of humour, though amidst the pearls of wisdom she gave to us and the patients there came the occasional reprimand.

To the newly qualified practitioner it was for making a stupid mistake. If the reprimand was directed at the patient it was for failing to help themselves by adopting a more positive attitude.

Shortly after this I was allowed again to experience the power of colour, when I unfortunately contracted shingles. After seeking medical advice I chose not to take the drugs prescribed but to treat myself. I worked with specific colours for the rash and with others to treat my whole body. In a very short time the rash disappeared with no neurological afterpain.

At the end of the year with Lily I incorporated colour therapy into my reflexology practice, treating patients with the therapy I felt would be most beneficial for them. After some years in practice, I was directed to integrate colour with reflexology and discovered that the combination of these two therapies was extremely powerful. Colour with reflexology frequently achieved what reflexology was unable to do alone. This led me to believe that colour could be an equally powerful tool if used with some of the other complementary therapies being practised.

In the years since my introduction to colour I have explored many of its other facets. Some of the information gleaned and experience gained from this I have incorporated into the teachings of the Oracle School of Colour, which I founded two years ago. I believe this school forms one of the branches of the colour school tree and, like all other schools, holds a part of the whole truth. What I have discovered from teaching is that my students are also my teachers. They frequently ask questions which lead me to undertake fresh research or they bring new ideas which we work with as a group. For all of this I thank them.

The purpose of this book is to share what I have learnt over the years with other colour practitioners, with those studying colour therapy and with those who simply wish to know more about the subject. For those studying colour therapy, especially my own students, this book has been written to serve as a teaching manual. If this is your first introduction to the subject, may I suggest that you first read my introductory book *A Piatkus Guide to Colour Healing* (Piatkus, 1999). This will give you a basic knowledge about colour and ideas on ways of helping yourself with it. The step-by-step treatment and some of the protection techniques given in this book are taken from Lily's work, which she was always happy to share with others. Some of the other topics covered, for example the aura and the metaphysical cause of certain diseases, may also be helpful to practitioners of other disciplines.

If after reading the book you feel that you would like to work with colour therapy, it is essential that you enrol at a colour school to study for a practitioner's diploma. It is not permissible to take the information given in this book and use it to give colour treatments. Colour can have adverse effects and therefore you need to know what you are doing. Information on colour practitioner training is given in the appendix.

Finally, I would like to thank Lily Cornford, to whom this book is dedicated, for teaching and watching over me during my training and first steps as a colour practitioner. Lily now lives in a nursing home and I am happy to say that I am still in contact with her.

Pauline Wills
July 1999

CHAPTER 1

THE NATURE OF LIGHT

FROM THE EARLIEST times man has been fascinated by the nature of light and colour. For centuries the appearance of the rainbow in the sky was a source of wonder. Many pondered on the reasons why the colours always appeared in the same order. From the time of Aristotle, philosophers tried to explain this phenomenon as the results of differing mixtures of light and darkness or shadow. They believed that white light mixed with a little shadow produced red, an assumption based on the red glow of sunset or sunrise appearing between the light of day and the darkness of night. A greater proportion of shadow added to light, they believed, produced green and a further increase in shadow would give rise to blue. But alas, these theories brought no closer understanding of the colour spectrum.

NEWTON'S DISCOVERIES

It was not until 1666, the year following the Great Plague, that a university student, Isaac Newton, laid the foundation for his exploration of the nature of light. Newton, then 23 years of age, had been intrigued by the French scientist René Descartes' account of his experiments with light, published in 1637. Descartes had observed how a prism could split white light into a spectrum of colour and concluded that the varying thickness of the prism was responsible for producing the different colours.

Newton decided to test Descartes' theory by designing a simple experiment of his own. He darkened one of the rooms in which he was staying, allowing only a thin beam of light to shine through a hole in one of the shutters.

On his workbench he arranged a triangular prism and a board on which to project light. When the beam of white sunlight shone through the prism, it produced the spectrum of red, orange, yellow, green, indigo and violet on the board as well as a change in the angle of the light. Newton then drilled a hole in the board in line with the red ray and placed a second prism behind the board. When the beam of red light passed through the second prism, it changed angle but failed to produce another spectrum. From this Newton concluded that white light was composed of different colours which the prism revealed rather than produced. To test his theory, Newton passed all the coloured rays which appeared through the first prism through a convex lens in order to focus the rays to pass through a second prism. What he found was the rays were refracted in the opposite direction and emerged as white light which when passed through a third prism, split again into the seven colours. By this experiment Newton conclusively demonstrated that white light is composed of the spectral colours (see below).

The angle change that Newton observed when he passed light through the prism became known as 'refraction'. This occurred because the prism altered the speed at which the light was travelling. This occurs when light is passed through any substance. One way to see refraction is to place a straw into a glass of water. The straw's shape will appear to change because the light rays bend with their reduction in speed upon entering the water (see page 10).

It is because each colour has a different angle of refraction that we are able to see the colour spectrum when light is passed through a prism, and this is the reason why the colours always appear in the same order. When we see the rainbow with the appearance of the sun after a storm, it is the raindrops that act like a prism, refracting the sun's light.

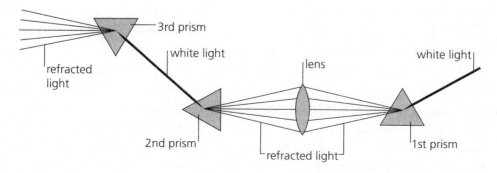

Newton's prism experiment

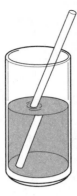

Refraction

Newton's concept of light was a stream of luminous corpuscles that travelled in a straight line with a different corpuscle for each colour. This explained many properties of light, such as reflection and refraction, but it could not explain the phenomenon of interference. This Newton experienced when he saw the colours in a soap bubble appearing in a different order from the rainbow colours. Sensing that this change in the order of colours had something to do with the thinness of the soap film which formed the bubble, he tried to produce a similar effect by shining a beam of light on to a very thin convex lens placed on a pane of glass. He found that where the light made contact with the centre of the lens and the pane of glass, darkness appeared, but radiating out from this were rings of faint blue, white, orange, red, dark purple and green. Although Newton had no explanation for their appearance, they became known as 'Newton's rings'.

INTERFERENCE

It was not until 1802 that the phenomenon that Newton had seen was understood. It became known as 'interference', the effect produced by the interaction of two or more different wave motions, and was demonstrated by the English physicist Thomas Young. In his experiment he used three screens placed at a set distance from each other. Into the first screen he cut a narrow slit and into the second screen he cut two narrow slits approximately 1mm apart. When he shone light through the single slit, the light spread out or defracted before passing through the two narrow slits, forming two sources of light which again defracted. When this light fell on to the third screen a central bright band of light appeared with alternate light and dark bands on either side. From this experiment Young learnt that as the light waves from the two slits spread out, they came into contact with each other. Where the crests or troughs of the waves coincided, known as 'constructive interference', they reinforced each other and produced bright bands of colour; where the crests coincided with the troughs, known as 'destructive interference', they cancelled each other out and created dark bands in the circle of light (see below). This phenomenon happens not only with light waves but also with sound and with water.

It was this experiment that made Young realise that light consisted of waves, but his findings and beliefs were not immediately accepted. Yet later Young's work on the wave theory of light led to the discovery that light has properties in common with other electromagnetic forms of radiation.

At the same time that Young was experimenting with 'interference' fringes, a surprising discovery was made about sunlight by William Hyde Wollaston. He found that instead of the sun's spectrum being a continuous band of light, it contained hundreds of narrow gaps where particular wavelengths were missing. It was not until the middle of the nineteenth century that the reason for this was found. The German physicist Gustav Kirchhoff discovered that these gaps occurred through the absorption by atoms of particular wavelengths of light. Although this was of major importance in showing that links existed between atoms and light, it was not until the twentieth century that a theory on the interaction of atoms and light emerged.

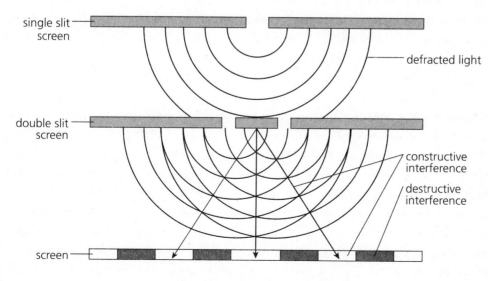

single slit screen

defracted light

double slit screen

constructive interference

destructive interference

screen

Young's double slit experiment

ATOMS AND LIGHT

This theory was originated by the German physicist Philipp Lenard. Alongside other physicists he was investigating the link between the wavelengths of light, the release of electrons and the energy they possessed. What was discovered was that certain metals emit electrons and electric current flows when light is absorbed by the metal, but the physicists could not explain why this happened. An explanation was not found until 1900 when the physicist Max Planck proposed that energy can be radiated or absorbed only in separate packets of energy (now called quanta). This revolutionary proposal marked the beginning of the quantum theory. In 1905 the German physicist Albert Einstein, said to be one of the greatest scientists of all time, extended this idea by suggesting that the quantum of energy emitted by an atom continues to exist as a concentrated packet of energy. In order to understand this and the nature of light, we need to know the structure of an atom.

An atom consists of a positively charged nucleus which is balanced by the negatively charged electrons orbiting it. The further the electrons are from the nucleus, the more energy they have; those closest to the nucleus have less energy. In most atoms there are many electrons and many different energy levels. Light frequencies, considered by Einstein to be a stream of energised particles which he called 'photons', are produced by the energy lost when an electron moves from one orbit to another. This is how light, heat and the invisible rays of the electromagnetic spectrum are produced by the atoms covering the surface of the sun.

If we imagine the orbits formed by the electrons as steps leading to the nucleus, an electron making a quantum leap, or moving up one step, would release a small amount of energy producing the long wavelengths manifesting red light. If the electron moves up seven steps, for example, it releases more energy, creating the short wavelengths of violet light. The steps in between form the quantum of wavelengths which produce the colours that fall between red and violet in the colour spectrum. From this theory, we can see that the long wavelengths of red light contain the least amount of energy, or fewest photons, and the short wavelengths of violet light the most (see opposite).

When light falls on an object, its photons interact with the atoms which make up the object. The electrons circulating within the atoms attract to

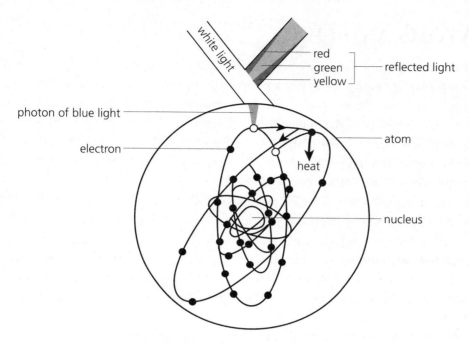

The structure of an atom

themselves the photons from the light that possess the desired energy to enable them to leap to the next orbit and release their energy as a small quantity of heat before returning to their original orbit. The photons which are not absorbed are reflected, giving the object its colour. For example, the chlorophyll in green vegetables absorbs all but the green photons which it reflects to give the vegetables their colour. The carotenoid pigment found in carrots absorbs the short wavelengths of blue, indigo and violet, and reflects red, orange, yellow and green, which produces the familiar orange colour of the carrot. This illustrates why a red vegetable or fruit is high in energy and a violet vegetable, for example, an aubergine, is low in energy.

All pigments are compounds which absorb and reflect particular wavelengths of light very efficiently. The absorption colours can be identified with a spectrometer. Some objects are capable of absorbing all the wavelengths constituting light and so appear black. On the other hand, objects that reflect all the wavelengths of light appear white. Those that absorb and reflect a proportion of each wavelength look grey.

Dyes and paints work on the same principle. For thousands of years only natural pigments were used to make dyes, which made some colours rare and expensive to buy, but with the discovery of synthetic pigments, the range of colours available has become limitless.

ELECTROMAGNETIC ENERGY

Electromagnetic energy originating from the sun ranges from the longest wavelengths, namely radio waves, to the shortest wavelengths, which are cosmic rays (see below). All of these rays are measured in metres and nanometres. The complete electromagnetic spectrum contains 60 or 70 octaves. All the electromagnetic energy travels at approximately 186,000 miles per second.

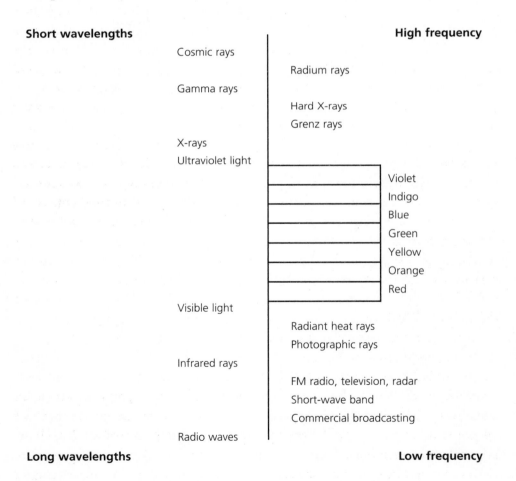

The electromagnetic spectrum

Except for visible light, all the electromagnetic rays are invisible to the human eye but are utilised by both science and medicine, sometimes beneficially but sometimes with detrimental results.

If we start by looking at radio waves, we find that their different wavebands work with radar, microwaves, ovens, television and radios. The short wave radio bands are used for diathermy, which is the application of electrical currents to produce heat in the deeper tissues of the body for the relief of rheumatism, arthritis and neuralgia. The low-level microwave radiation used in microwave ovens rapidly changes the alignment of water molecules to heat up food. I believe that this has a detrimental effect on the nutritional value of the food being heated.

Moving on from radio waves, we come to infrared waves, which are produced by anything that is hot. Infrared waves include photographic and radiant heat waves; they have the power to travel great distances and to penetrate heavy atmospheres. The photographic rays react with photographic plates to take pictures which the human eye has difficulty seeing. The radiant heat rays are used for drying and these can be emitted by steam radiators, electric heaters and infrared lamps.

Following infrared comes visible light. This part of the spectrum is visible to human beings because our eyes contain nerve endings called rods and cones that are sensitive to a particular range of wavelengths. The rods are responsible for night vision and the cones for distinguishing the colours of light. These are measured in nanometres. The measurement for each spectral colour is:

Red light:	627–780 nanometres
Orange light:	589–627 nanometres
Yellow light:	556–589 nanometres
Green light:	495–556 nanometres
Blue light:	436–495 nanometres
Violet light:	380–436 nanometres

Passing from visible light, we come to the invisible waves of ultraviolet which carry more energy than visible light and are produced by very hot objects. Ultraviolet is divided into three wavebands: A, B and C. Waveband A is able to pass through most types of glass, produces slight erythema (reddening of the skin) and causes certain materials to fluoresce while bringing about a photochemical reaction in others. It is used in various industrial processes and in UV lamps. Waveband B has both an erythemal and a pigmenting effect on the human skin. Its ability to form vitamin D in the body aids the calcium process and helps prevent or cure rickets. This makes its use mainly therapeutic. Waveband C has a germicidal effect but can cause erythema and conjunctivitis. Certain materials fluoresce when exposed to this ray.

As the wavelengths become shorter we come into X-rays. These include Grenz rays (which are soft X-rays) and hard X-rays. Hard X-rays are those which destroy the cells of the human body and are used in the treatment of malignant tumours. In industry they are used to detect flaws in metal. Soft X-rays are able to penetrate the soft parts of our bodies but they cannot pass through bone, enabling them to be used to photograph the skeletal system. They are also widely used by the medical profession for diagnostic purposes but overdoses can cause anaemia, roentgen sickness and carcinomas. Unfortunately X-rays are cumulative in the physical body. If used during pregnancy, they can cause serious deformities to the foetus.

Nearing the end of the scale are the gamma or radium rays discovered by Pierre and Marie Curie at the beginning of the twentieth century. Gamma rays have very short wavelengths and are a form of radioactivity. They carry a large amount of energy and are capable of penetrating metals and concrete. Gamma rays are used in the treatment of malignant tumours but because they are highly dangerous and can be damaging to health, they are very carefully monitored.

At the top of the electromagnetic scale, with the shortest wavelengths, are cosmic rays. These are high energy radiation, containing tiny particles of atomic nuclei as well as some electrons and gamma rays. Cosmic radiation bombards the Earth's atmosphere from remote regions of space.

When I studied the electromagnetic spectrum there was one question which constantly came into my mind. That question was: if science and medicine appreciate how the invisible rays of the electromagnetic spectrum affect both humans and objects and have utilised these rays in both industry and medicine, how can they say that the visible part of the spectrum, namely light, does not affect us? It was not until I studied visible light and started to work as a colour practitioner that I proved for myself that the colours constituting light do affect us and are a powerful medium in healing. I am happy to report that allopathic medicine is now looking at the therapeutic effects of light and starting to utilise it.

HOW COLOUR IS PERCEIVED

Colours are perceived through the eyes. Sight, as we know it, has been developed during the course of evolution from a variety of simple photosensory cells.

The simple or complex structure of each species' eyes determine which colours, if any, it is able to see. Many primitive animals, such as worms and a few insects, possess simple organs of sight called ocelli. These ocelli have a primitive lens which focuses light on to a very simple retina, allowing such creatures to distinguish between darkness and light. As life evolved, most insects and crustacea developed compound eyes resembling the many facets which form a diamond. Each facet consists of a minute lens which focuses on one part of the field of vision and transmits light to a small number of photosensitive cells which comprise an ommatidium. Signals from the receptors in each ommatidium are transmitted directly to the brain, which builds up a picture of the whole field of vision. It is thought that insects with compound eyes are not sensitive to the red end of the spectrum but highly sensitive to green, blue, violet and ultraviolet.

Experiments have shown that colour vision is not apparent in fish which live in the murky waters near the sea bed, but that it does exist in fish which live near to the surface of the sea. In birds, scientists have found that most are partially blind to blue but see red with remarkable clarity. Behavioural experiments to test whether the various species of animals can see colour suggest that dogs only have rudimentary colour vision and that cats can see colour only if the coloured surface is above a certain critical size, but that tortoises have good colour vision.

Vertebrate animals, which include man, have the most sophisticated eyes, in which a single lens directs light on to an array of photosensitive cells, similar to the lens of a camera focusing light on to a film. Anthropologists believe that early man was able to see only in black and white, with colour vision developing at a later era.

The eyes of human beings are complex and thought by Jacob Liberman (see page 31) to be an extension of the brain. The eyeball is a sphere approximately 2.5cm in diameter and is divided into two compartments by the crystalline lens and its associated structure, which is suspended just behind the iris. The larger of these compartments is situated behind the lens and is filled with a transparent fluid which ensures the eyeball maintains its correct shape. The anterior chamber, filled with aqueous humour, forms the front part of the eyeball, bounded by the cornea in front and the lens and iris behind. Between these two chambers lies the ciliary body containing the ciliary muscles and ducts for draining the aqueous humour. The remaining structure of the eye consists of the sclera, which is the outer coat of the eye and seen as the white of the eye; the cornea, which is the transparent curved anterior part of the eyeball that helps to focus the light source; the choroid, the middle vascular coat of the eye composed largely of interlaced blood vessels providing nutrition to the eye; the iris, which is the pigmented continuation of the choroid coat in front of the lens; the pupil, the circular hole in front of the lens surrounded by the iris; the macula, an area of the retina where light focuses on densely packed cells, the fovea, which forms the centre of the macula; and the retina, a very thin, light-sensitive tissue which lines the back of the eye, curving forward like a deep rounded cup (see below). The nerves from the retina join to form the optic or eleventh cranial nerve.

In human beings the retina is formed from photoreceptor cells known as rods or cones. There are approximately 120,000,000 rods found throughout the retina but none in the area of the fovea. The rods contain the visual pigment rhodopsin and are most sensitive to blue/green light of 505 nanometres.

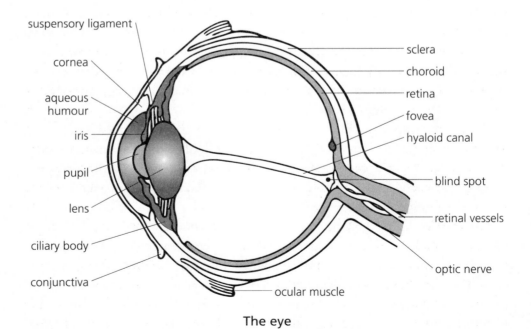

The eye

They work in dim light to produce night vision. The cones, numbering approximately 6,000,000, are responsible for colour vision. There are three types of cones containing three different types of pigment which are sensitive to the spectral hues of red, green and blue, with a predominance of red and green cones. These are concentrated in the fovea, which is responsible for acute vision. When the red and green cones are equally stimulated, the sensation of yellow is generated. The blue cones are found sparsely scattered among the rods with maybe a few contained in the fovea. All three types of cones have a broad absorption spectra ranging between 400 and 700 nanometres.

When light falls on the eye it is refracted by the cornea, entering the eye chamber through the pupil. The iris, surrounding the pupil, will dilate in bright light and constrict in dim light to alter the size of the pupil to admit the right amount of light. The light then passes through the lens, whose shape is determined by the ciliary muscles, and focuses a sharp, inverted image on the retina. Here light is absorbed by the photoreceptors constituting the rods and cones. Any light not absorbed by the photoreceptors is absorbed by a layer of cells which line the back of the retina. The light absorbed by the photoreceptors is translated into patterns of electrical signals which are transmitted through a complex process to the head of the optic nerve which then transmits them to the visual cortex at the back of the brain.

There are two other pathways for light, the first of which little is known. This runs from the nerve ganglion cell layer of the retina direct to the hypothalamus. The hypothalamus and the pituitary gland work together to control most of the other endocrine glands in the physical body. As a result, the hypothalamus is able to control through the pituitary the functions in the body which are known to be influenced by the perception of light. These include body temperature, metabolism, water regulation and sexual and reproductive functions. The pituitary and hypothalamus also control our sleeping and behavioural patterns, appetite and the balance of the autonomic nervous system. The hypothalamus also houses the body's biological clock.

Light entering the eye affects the autonomic nervous system via the second non-visual route which connects the eye to the pineal gland. A small number of nerve fibres leaving the eye are diverted along the inferior accessory optic tract and it is these nerve fibres which allow nerve impulses from the eye to be transmitted from the brain to the spinal cord. The impulses leave the spinal cord, just below the neck, to enter the superior cervical nerve ganglion of the sympathetic nervous system, from where they travel by a set route back to the pineal gland.

The pineal gland is frequently described as the 'light meter' of the body, receiving information from the environment about light and darkness by way of the eyes. This gland's secretions are determined by the number of sympathetic nerve impulses reaching it and these impulses are either suppressed or stimulated by the nerve transmission from the eyes when the retina reacts to light.

Both of these non-visual routes show us how important it is for the eyes to absorb natural daylight. I personally believe that a number of today's diseases are caused through light malnutrition and that our general health will improve greatly if we allow ourselves at least 30 minutes outdoors a day without wearing glasses or contact lenses.

Throughout history there have been many other ways of using light and colour for therapeutic purposes and it is to these that we shall turn now.

CHAPTER 2

THE HISTORY OF COLOUR THERAPY

LIGHT IS DERIVED from the sun, whose warmth and light are essential to sustain all life-forms. For this reason the sun and the gods ascribed to it have been worshipped by man throughout the ages. In ancient Egypt, the sun at its zenith was seen as the embodiment of the god Ra, whilst the rising sun was attributed to Horus and the setting sun to Osiris. The ancient Greeks related the sun to Apollo and to the eye of Zeus whilst on the other side of the world the Incas depicted it in human form with a radiant disc of gold for the face. The sun god of the Maya was Ahau Kin, who could appear in youthful or aged aspects and between sunset and sunrise he was believed to journey through the underworld as the jaguar god. In Hinduism the sun is 'The Vivifier' and for Christians it symbolises God the Father, ruler and sustainer of the universe, radiating both light and love.

Dante wrote: 'There is no visible thing in all the world more worthy to serve as a symbol of God than the sun, which illuminates with visible light, first itself, then all the celestial and mundane bodies.'

In most traditions, the sun is known as the Universal Father and is connected to the right eye. The left eye and Universal Mother are ascribed to the moon. The sun is responsible for ordering people's lives through the rhythms of the seasons and of the day and night. Early man greatly benefited from the sun's healing rays because he spent most of his waking hours outside hunting and working. After sunset, he retired to the back of his cave to sleep until dawn. Unfortunately our modern way of life keeps us indoors for the majority of the day, depriving us of the natural sunlight which is so essential to health.

For many cultures, the solstices and equinoxes of the sun are of major importance. The equinoxes are the two points each year when days and nights are equal in length and the sun is at zero declination. In the northern hemisphere these occur in the spring, around 21 March, and in the autumn, around 22 September. In the southern hemisphere, the seasons are reversed. The solstices occur when the sun appears to 'stand still' at its highest or lowest declination in the sky, producing the longest day and shortest night in the summer and the shortest day and longest night in the winter. At the summer solstice, around 1 June in the northern hemisphere, the sun appears at its highest declination in the sky because the Earth is at the lowest point in its orbit; at the winter solstice, around 22 December in the northern hemisphere, the sun appears at its lowest declination in the sky because the Earth is at the highest point in its orbit. The winter solstice is purported to be the 'door of the gods', symbolising the ascent and growing power of the sun. The summer solstice refers to the 'door of men' and is linked to the descent and waning power of the sun.

In many civilisations, light is associated with the manifestation of divinity and represents truth and direct knowledge, ultimately leading to a state of enlightenment, a state of wholeness. To ancient man, light was seen as sustaining life. Enlightenment was therefore synonymous with health which incorporated body, mind and spirit. In order to reach this state of wholeness, it was believed that these three aspects of their being had to become harmonious with each other. This concept is still upheld today by complementary therapists.

In ancient times, magic and ritual played a large part in healing. Magicians believed that they could achieve this state of enlightenment and bring it to those who were sick by 'bringing down the light', transferring and reflecting its power. This belief created a link between magic, religion and medicine.

EARLY USES OF LIGHT AND COLOUR

According to material channelled by Frank Alper and published in his books on Atlantis, light and colour were used by the Atlanteans in healing (*Exploring Atlantis*, vols 1, 2 and 3, Arizona Metaphysical Society, 1981). Alper speaks of circular temples around whose circumference were healing rooms. The roofs of these temples were made from interlocking crystals which refracted the sunlight, filling the temple with the spectral colours. The doors to the healing rooms were apparently designed to resonate to the required colour frequency, and these rooms were used for childbirth, healing relationships and to aid the transition from earthly life to spiritual life through death. The Atlanteans are also thought to have incorporated specific geometric patterns, formed with the aid of crystals, into their healing techniques. These, they believed, amplified the vibrational energy of the colours being used.

In ancient Egypt, every aspect of health or illness was associated with a deity. Ra the sun god held the highest place in the pantheon, while Isis was worshipped as a healing goddess with temples dedicated to her healing power. Among other supernatural healers were Hathor, mistress of heaven and protector of women in childbirth. The two most important healing divinities were Thoth and Imhotep. Thoth became a patron god both of physicians and of scribes and the use of colour in healing was attributed to him. In Egyptian treatments, religious and magical gestures played a vital role. Incantations were used to drive out demons and supplications made to the gods to protect patients from harmful spirits. The healers used colour through herbs and plants, salves and dyes alongside coloured minerals and metals such as copper, carbon and antimony, which was also high in the paints used for beautifying women's eyes. Antimony was thought to have antiseptic properties which prevented eye disease.

Archaeologists have discovered that the Egyptians, like the Atlanteans, had individual healing rooms built into their lavishly decorated temples. These rooms were constructed in such a way that when the sun entered them, its rays were dissipated into the colours of the spectrum. Those coming for healing were 'colour diagnosed' and then put into the room which radiated the prescribed colour.

Magic, colour and healing were also linked in India. India is a country alive with colour. Hinduism is one of its oldest living religions, having evolved over a period of 4,000 years and its ancient teachings have formed the foundations of traditional Indian Ayurvedic (knowledge of life) medicine. Hindus believe that all the gods they worship affect health and illness. The *Atharva-Veda*, which forms part of the *Vedas*, a collection of ancient hymns and prayers, contains a collection of spells and incantations to combat disease, injuries, fertility and insanity. Methods of diagnosis included magical as well as rational approaches. Treatment included the use of minerals and gemstones, which were believed to be a concentration of the seven cosmic rays.

To this present day Ayurvedic medicine works with gemstones, relating onyx to ultraviolet light, cat's eye to infrared, ruby to red, pearl to orange, coral to yellow, emerald to green, topaz to blue, diamond to indigo and sapphire to violet. These gems were always examined through a prism to ascertain their true cosmic colour as it was believed that the manifested colour was not always the true essence of the stone.

Classical Chinese medicine was based primarily on works ascribed to three legendary emperors: Fu Hs, responsible for the composition of the yang and yin lines; She Nung, the Red Emperor, who compiled the first medical herbal; and Yi Hsiung, the Yellow Emperor, who compiled the great medical compendium, the *Nei Ching* (Canon of Medicine). According to this, there were five methods of treatment: cure the spirit, nourish the body, give medication, treat the whole body and use acupuncture and moxibustion. Colour was used in the form of herbs, minerals and salves.

At this present time colour has been reintroduced to this ancient art of healing in the form of 'colourpuncture'. This involves administering the correct colour, in the form of light, to the acupuncture points. This method was founded and developed by scientist Peter Mandel. He found that by focusing coloured light on acupuncture points on the skin powerful healing impulses were triggered in the physical and energy bodies.

Colour was used alongside sound in ancient Greece. The philosopher Pythagoras established a philosophical medical centre based on Orphic mysticism, which included a belief in reincarnation and asceticism. The Pythagoreans worked with the science of numbers and established scientific theories of sound and musical octaves which they used alongside colour in their healing methods. Colour and sound have a great affinity with each other. Both are vibrational energy and each spectral colour with its varying shades and hues can be intimately linked to a specific sound. Added to this, the Pythagoreans taught the importance of diet, exercise and medication.

Another Greek physician, Hippocrates, born on the island of Cos and said to be the father of modern medicine, has had many stories written about him, some believed to be true and some false. The most widely known document associated with him is the Hippocratic Oath which contains both affirmations and prohibitions. He is believed to have worked alongside the Greek system which explained the mechanism of illness in terms of four basic humours or bodily fluids. These are blood (red), which is connected to the heart; yellow bile, associated with the spleen; black bile, arising in the brain;

and white phlegm, deriving from the liver. When these were kept in equilibrium, harmony and health were established. It has also been suggested that Hippocrates was an alchemist and therefore employed both colour and magic in his healing techniques. These would have included the use of flowers, plasters, ointments and minerals.

Alongside the use of colour, treatment by sunlight (heliotherapy) was a common practice among the Greeks and Romans who, it has been suggested, were the first to write down both its theory and practice. Herodotus is purported to be the father of this treatment. The Greek city of Heliopolis was famous for its healing temples which were designed to refract sunlight into the spectral colours in similar ways to both the Atlantean and Egyptian temples.

THE CHRISTIAN ERA

During the first five centuries of the Christian era medical practices involving colour, chants and worship of various gods were deemed pagan. This drove such practices underground, where the ancient knowledge was passed on by word of mouth. Due to this, much of the Greek and Roman writings on holistic medical procedures were lost. In Judaic thought, disease had long been equated with sin's punishment or with divine disfavour and the early Christian Church did little to discourage this belief, teaching that the appropriate response was to suffer until a cure was brought about by grace and divine intervention.

In the seventh century, the new evangelical religion of Islam was moved to preserve what medical writings still remained and to translate them into Arabic and later into Latin. The most frequently translated works were those of Aristotle, Hippocrates and the Greek physician Galen.

One of the early translators was Avicenna, an outstanding physician and the restorer of colour to medicine. Avicenna was born in Persia and reputed to be a child prodigy. He is said to have mastered the Koran by the age of 10. He was intrigued by the ideas of Aristotle and wrote a scientific encyclopaedia at 21 years of age. The most renowned of his approximately 100 books was *The Canon*, upon which untold numbers of translators, teachers, students and practitioners based their medical ideas and procedures. In this *Canon* Avicenna made reference to his own ideas and findings on the use of colour in treatment. These included the adverse effects that colour can produce. His three main treatment colours were red, blue and yellow. He noted that red increased blood pressure whilst blue lowered it. Yellow, he proclaimed, reduced inflammation and pain.

During the Middle Ages mysticism again became prevalent with the incantation of chants being practised in the presence of a diseased individual, in the preparation of drugs and during surgery. Astrology was also given great weight. During the later part of the Middle Ages possession by devils was thought to be related to specific illnesses and amulets were worn to ward off these and all harmful spirits.

Although medical treatment in the Middle Ages appears to be a bizarre combination of science and mysticism, it was derived from the redefinition of the classical conception of humours. With this redefinition colour was again brought into play through the administration of herbs, plant extracts and salves. Alongside these, the less holistic method of bloodletting was practised.

During the Renaissance, medical practices made great strides, with physicians being well versed in physics and astronomy and having a growing interest in magic. The study of Hippocrates and open-minded observation of natural phenomena were increasing.

One outstanding healer of this period was Theophrastus Bombastus von Hohenheim, or Paracelsus. Paracelsus was born near Zurich, held a doctor's degree and developed considerable interest in alchemy, astrology and the occult sciences. He took his considerable interest in alchemy to heart and in applying this to the treatment of disease, earned himself the title 'Father of Pharmacology'. He believed that diseases were caused by the influences of the stars and planets upon the astral body of man. His great interest in alchemy led to his use of colour in his medical practice. This he administered with light, herbs and minerals.

The seventeenth century, the 'Age of the Scientific Revolution', represented a major turning-point in the history of science. Instead of scientists asking why things occurred, they turned to enquiring how things happened. But therapy was still mainly a continuation of the past in terms of purging and using drugs derived from plants, minerals and animal parts.

Great medical advances were made in the understanding of anatomy in the nineteenth century through the dissection of corpses and surgical procedures together with the use of drugs. With the advent of this so-called 'modern medicine', the concept of treating the whole person was lost. Science and medical practices became united, placing emphasis on the physical body, and the diseases from which it suffered. These new concepts excluded the spiritual, emotional and mental aspects. With their disappearance, colour also became excluded.

Towards the middle of the nineteenth century, however, treatment with sunlight was reintroduced by Jakob Lorber. Information on the application techniques were detailed in his book *The Healing Power of Sunlight* first published in 1851 in German (English translation, Gerhard Hansville and Franco Gallo, Merkur Publishing Inc., 1997). Lorber maintained that the information given in this book came directly from God. He advocates that any part of the body suffering disease should be exposed to the sun's rays, alongside the taking of clear, clean, sun-infiltrated spring water. The importance of diet is also emphasised.

Lorber describes the solarisation of saclose pellets and how these should be stored to keep their potency. He gives techniques for solarising sulphuric or pure sea salt, which he claims is an excellent remedy for bone fractures. He maintains that for good results this should be administered to a patient on a spoon made from gold or the finest silver. He believed that solarised salt placed on the tongue of a person near to death would completely restore them, providing they were not too emaciated, but if complete recovery were not possible then the person's life would be extended for a while. He also contends that solarising the blood of a lamb or healthy calf until the blood turns into a reddish brown powder makes an excellent remedy for lung disease and haemorrhage. Towards the end of the book he gives sunlight remedies for specific ailments, including malignant tumours, and the preparation of sunlight tinctures. Although solarised water and solarised placebos are used today in colour therapy, more advanced methods have been developed.

Another pioneer of sunlight treatment, perhaps the most prominent, was the Danish physician Niels Ryberg Finsen (1860–1904). He was the first to develop light treatment scientifically, using artificial light, particularly the carbon arc. His use of the carbon arc started in 1892 for the treatment of skin tuberculosis (*lupus vulgaris*). He observed that this condition was more prevalent in winter and deduced that sunlight played an important role in this disease. For his many years of work in this field and his reported miraculous cures of many people, he received the Nobel Prize in 1903 and became known as the 'Father of Photobiology'.

The most acclaimed person for using heliotherapy on a large scale in

Switzerland was Dr Augustus Rollier (*La Care de Soleil*, 1903). He used it in sanatoria for the prevention and treatment of tuberculosis. When he first presented evidence of his cures at a medical congress in Paris he was ridiculed by the audience. Undeterred, he continued his work, setting up 36 clinics for treatment. He believed in the healing power of the sun and took photographs before and after treatment to support his claims.

THE REDISCOVERY OF COLOUR

During this time, practitioners using the direct rays of the sun in healing started again to look at the colours which constituted this light. Two of the early pioneers in this field were Dr Seth Pancoast and Dr Edwin Babitt. Pancoast published a book entitled *Blue & Red Lights* (J.M. Stoddart & Co., 1877) in which he describes the use of blue and red glass filters in his treatments. He believed that the red ray accelerated the nervous system and the blue ray relaxed it. His great interest lay in cabalistic teachings and the wisdom of ancient philosophers. It was upon these teachings that he based some of his colour-related knowledge.

In 1878 Dr Edwin Babitt published his outstanding book *The Principles of Light and Colour* (self published). A great deal of his work involved the three primary colours, red, yellow and blue. He believed that red was the centre of heat and the ruling colour of hydrogen, yellow was the centre of luminosity and blue was the centre of electricity and the ruling colour of oxygen. He administered colour to his patients in a cabinet that he had invented, called the 'Thermoline', which made use of natural sunlight. The Thermoline was later remodelled so that the source of light came from what Babitt described as an 'electric arc'. With this latest model he used a 'chromodisc' to which he fitted coloured filters. This enabled him to project colour on to specific parts of the body. Coupled with this he used solarised water. To solarise the water he fitted a small glass bottle with a 'chromo lens' (developed for this purpose) of the colour required and hung it in the sunlight. When the water was ready he gave it to his patients to drink.

During the early part of the twentieth century, investigations into colour were being carried out by the occultist, philosopher, teacher and religious leader Rudolf Steiner, who believed that colour was a living entity and that each colour bore a spiritual significance. Steiner maintained that colour would play a very important part in medicine in the twenty-first century. He believed that illness was caused through the separation of earthly conscious-ness from higher perception and that this separation could be healed through art. The main colours he worked with were red, blue, yellow, green, white, black and peach blossom. These he divided into two categories. He called red, blue and yellow 'the active colours' and white, black, green and peach blossom 'the image colours'. He related these to mathematical form, believ-ing that form had the power to amplify the healing effect of colour. His work is carried on today in the Rudolf Steiner schools which he founded.

Unlike Steiner, Max Luscher, a former Professor of Psychology at Basle University and author of *The Luscher Colour Test* (translated and edited by Ian Scott, Pan Books, 1971) believes that colour can treat and determine both physical and psychological illnesses. He bases his belief on the theory that a person's preference for certain colours is directly related to the 'emo-tional value' of these colours. The colours people prefer, dislike or are indif-ferent to, he believes, are indicators of basic personality traits. His colour theories originate from the lifestyle of early man, whose life he believes was controlled by the light of day or the darkness of night. During daylight hours man was active, thereby increasing his metabolic rate and glandular secre-tions. At night the reverse occurred, inducing a state of peace and relaxation. He therefore associated dark blue, the colour of night, with quietness and passivity, and yellow, the colour of day, with hope and activity. Luscher fur-ther believes that primitive man spent his waking hours either hunting and attacking, and this he attributed to the colour red, or being hunted and defending himself, which he associated with the colour green.

Luscher's colour theories were supported by a Russian scientist S. V. Krakov, who later proved that red stimulates the sympathetic part of the nervous system and blue stimulates the parasympathetic part (see 'Colour Vision and the Nervous System', *Journal of the Optical Society of America*, June 1942).

Two of the great twentieth-century innovators for colour therapy were Dinshah P. Ghadiali and Dr Harry Riley Spitler. Ghadiali, born in India in 1873, had no medical training, but was awarded four honorary medical degrees for his work and research into colour. In 1934 he published his three-volume work, *The Spectro-Chrome Metry Encyclopedia* (vols 1, 2 and 3, Spectro-Chrome Institute, Malaga, NJ, 1939) which constituted a home colour training course. Ghadiali was well versed in electricity, mathematics and physics, and believed that sound, light, colour magnetism and heat were all the same energy, the only difference being their vibrational frequency. With his scientific background in physics and chemistry, he set out to formulate a scientific approach for the application of colour to the human body. He related colour and vibration to the physiology of the human body, believing that no elements are pure but that they themselves are compounds which do not possess a single or pure spectrum.

To apply the 12 colours he worked with, Ghadiali invented two machines to transmit these colours through slides. The first, which was called the 'graduate spectro-chrome', contained a 2,000-watt concentrated bulb, was driven by a motor and had built into it revolving coloured slides which were housed in an aluminium slide carrier. The second machine was the aluminium spectro-chrome, which he invented for family home use. This contained a 1,000-watt bulb and a sealed semaphore slide carrier which contained the Dinshah-attuned colour wave slides. It had its own stand and an automatic time switch, and came with a spectro-chrome home guide.

Although Ghadiali's work has not been scientifically proven, he has many supporters amongst whom is Dr Kate Baldwin, a senior surgeon working in America. She claims that she can produce quicker and more accurate results with colour than with any or all of the other methods combined, and with less strain on the patient. She also believes that if colour treatment is given before and after surgery the healing process is quicker.

Dr Harry Riley Spitler, a medical doctor and optometrist, was responsible for a system of colour treatment which he called 'Syntonics'. In 1933 he founded the College of Syntonic Optometry, which defined syntonics as 'the branch of ocular science dealing with selected portions of the visible spectrum' (*The Syntonic Principle*, College of Syntonic Optometry, 1941). Having studied the work of his predecessors and researched the use of colour in therapy in the sanatorium which he managed, he started to work by applying light directly through the eyes, with very positive results. This led him to experiment further with rabbits. These animals showed abnormal changes when subjected to certain colours. This convinced Spitler that light entering the eyes played an important role in the functioning of both the endocrine system and the autonomic nervous system. This in turn led him to believe that this system of treatment was able to change a person's vision due to the eyes' dependence on the nervous system. When treating in this way, he took into consideration the physical, mental and emotional make up of the person, realising that if a therapy were to succeed, the whole person had to be treated and not just the complaint. Unlike Ghadiali's, Spitler's treatments involved working with 31 different filter combinations.

In 1977, Jacob Liberman, an optometrist in the USA, heard of the work of Spitler and attended one of the courses held at the College of Syntonic Optometry. He purchased their equipment and carried on where Spitler had left off. Through his work he has become one of the pioneers in the field of therapeutic light treatment and has developed what he calls 'ocular photo-therapy'. For this treatment he constructed a machine which employs 20 coloured filters, evaluated to span the entire visible spectrum, and thought to be the most advanced machine of its kind for healing with light. Like Spitler, Liberman advocates that in order for a person to be made whole, the mental, emotional and spiritual aspects have to be taken into consideration alongside the physical. He also teaches that the eyes are the mirrors which radiate the light contained within each person. As the individual works towards wholeness, their inner light expands and radiates through their eyes. He has published two books, *Light: Medicine of The Future* (Bear & Co., 1991) and *Take Off Your Glasses and See* (Thorsons, 1995) which explain his work.

As Liberman so rightly says, we are beings of light and therefore need the natural light that radiates from the sun if we are to maintain our health.

Another pioneer who worked towards proving this was John Ott. Ott was a banker by profession but worked with time-lapse photography as a hobby. This led him to discover the importance of ultraviolet light for the healthy growth of plants. He later carried out controlled experiments with mice and, as with the plants, found that those living in natural daylight lived longer than those living under artificial light which eliminated the ultraviolet ray.

Ott himself suffered from arthritis. One day he broke his glasses, which necessitated him working outdoors without them. Over a period of one week, he found that his arthritis improved, allowing him to walk without his cane. From this and other experiments that he carried out, he deduced that only approximately 2 per cent of ultraviolet light passes through glass. As his own health had dramatically improved without his glasses, he realised that full-spectrum light, absorbed through the eyes, is essential for human health (see his book, *Health and Light*, Ariel Press, 1973).

In 1934, following on from the work of Ghadiali and Spitler, Dr Emmitt Knott and Dr Virgil Hancock published their findings concerning the use of an instrument invented by Dr Knott called the Haemo-Irradiation Machine.

The purpose of this machine was to irradiate a small amount of blood extracted from a patient with ultraviolet light before reinfusing it back into the patient. The name given to the therapy was 'ultraviolet irradiated blood retransfusions' (UVIBR). The physicians' published findings included the successful treatment of viral infections, peritonitis and advanced toxaemia. Apparently this form of treatment worked where drug treatment had failed. It was used in Germany, the United States and the Soviet Union up until the mid fifties. It was then abandoned for various reasons until the mid seventies, when it was reintroduced into medicine and elaborated upon in the Soviet Union. In the mid eighties another method of photomodification was developed, involving 'intravenous visible laser light irradiation of blood' (ILIB).

Today, both these forms of treatment are being carried out in Russia by Professor Kira Samoilova PhD. Samoilova graduated from the Leningrad University Biological Faculty in 1957 before completing her post-graduate studies at the Institute of Cytology of the Russian Academy of Sciences in St Petersburg where she now works. Her initial studies were focused on structural-functional changes in animal cells under the effect of UVC radiation. In the 1980s she became actively involved in scientific substantiation for new methods of phototherapy in both conventional and veterinary medicine. She published over 150 papers detailing the results of these investigations and a book entitled *Effect of UV Radiation on the Cell* (Nauka, Leningrad, 1967). She is currently chief editor of seven collective monographs in the fields of photobiology and photomedicine.

MODERN LIGHT TREATMENT

At this present time several forms of light treatment are being used by the medical profession. Blue light is being used with jaundiced premature babies. Studies done in the 1960s suggested that blue light was able to rid the infant's body of bilirubin that the immature liver was unable to cope with. Prior to using blue light, the infant was subjected to a blood transfusion which sometimes proved fatal. (For further information see J. R. Lacy, *Neonatal Jaundice and Phototherapy*, Paediatric Clinics of North America 19, 1972).

Ultraviolet light, first used in the 1990s is still utilised for skin problems such as acne and psoriasis. We frequently hear of the detrimental effects of over exposure to ultraviolet light, one being skin cancer. This theory is correct and even more care should be taken now that the ozone layer surrounding the Earth is being destroyed. But, having said this, we still need ultraviolet light for our well-being. To obtain this does not mean sitting in the sun for endless hours. It can be absorbed through the eyes, provided that spectacles and contact lenses are removed, by walking in the shade.

Seasonal Affective Disorder (SAD) is another condition which is now being treated with full-spectrum light. This disorder, discovered by Dr Norman Rosenthal (*Seasons of the Mind*, Bantam, 1989), himself a sufferer, starts with the onset of autumn and disappears in spring. It is caused by high levels of melatonin (a hormone secreted by the pineal gland), in the blood during daylight hours. This results in lethargy, depression and a craving for carbohydrates. I always think of melatonin as our hibernatory hormone. When darkness falls, its secretion is increased, inducing sleep. When dawn breaks, the light of the new day triggers the pineal gland to decrease the amount produced. During the winter months, with their minimal daylight hours, an overproduction of this hormone can be secreted into the bloodstream. Treatment for this condition requires sitting in front of a SAD light box, housing up to six full-spectrum, flicker-free fluorescent tubes, for anything from half an hour to three hours each day. The time factor depends upon the strength of the light emitted from the SAD box. This treatment achieves what a normal sunny summer day would achieve – a decrease in the hormonal production of the pineal gland.

Laser Light

In 1960 an American physicist built a machine that was able to produce a beam of very pure, concentrated light. This became known as a laser, which stands for 'Light Amplification by Stimulated Emission of Radiation'. Unlike the light given off by atoms, which is emitted at random, making it a mixture of many types of waves, the light produced by a laser is of a single wavelength and all the waves are in phase with each other, or 'coherent', allowing a very high level of energy to be projected as a parallel beam.

Laser light is produced by feeding energy into a solid liquid or gas. The type of liquid or gas used determines the type of laser produced. The three great advantages of lasers are their potency, their speed of action and their ability to focus on an extremely small area. For these reasons they have allowed great advances to be made in microsurgery, particularly fibreoptic endoscopy.

The two main uses of lasers in surgery are the endoscopic photocoagulation of bleeding vessels and the incision of tissue. The first of these uses the argon laser, which produces the visible green wavelength, and the latter uses the carbon dioxide laser, which produces an infrared beam.

Lasers have important applications in ophthalmology in the treatment of detached retinas and proliferative retinopathy (a condition associated with diabetes). They are also used in dermatology in the treatment of pigmented lesions, in the obliteration of 'port wine stains', in the removal of small benign tumours such as verrucas and in the removal of tattoos.

A treatment pioneered by Professor Endre Mester at Semmelweis University, Budapest, is the use of soft laser light for the elimination of pain for burn victims and for accelerating the healing of wounds. It has been reported that soft laser light can halve the healing time and reduce scar tissue.

Polarised light treatment has been developed in Budapest by Dr Marta Fenyo. Dr Fenyo is a biophysicist, laser specialist and inventor. With the aid of John Stephenson, an ergonomics consultant, physics genius and inventor, she believes that she has made a breakthrough in medicine with this light.

Initially, Dr Fenyo was working alongside Professor Endre Mester, researching the effect of soft lasers on leg ulcers, bedsores and varicose problems. The results they were getting were excellent, but the difficulty was the lack of money to buy the necessary equipment to treat the thousands of people suffering these complaints. Fenyo then started to experiment to find out which component in laser light was responsible for the healing process. The answer she came up with was polarised light. She then used every resource possible to prove her theory.

In the meantime, John Stephenson had been asked by the UK Ministry of Defence to improve the working environment of their civil servants. Examining the work conducted by Dr Fritz Hollwich on people's biological response to fluorescent light and full-spectrum light and Professor Blackwell's research of polarised artificial light, he came to the conclusion that the most beneficial light is that which is both polarised and full spectrum. Whilst attending a health fair, Stephenson came across a leaflet advertising the work of Fenyo, which resulted in their meeting.

From the work of these two people came the discovery that polarised light boosts the immune system and has a dramatic healing effect on varicose ulcers. In experiments carried out on mice infected with cancers, Fenyo found that treatment with polarised light increased their life expectancy and in some cases allowed them to live out their full life span. From dogs dying of cancer, she extracted a tiny portion of blood, treated it with polarised light and then reinfused it. The results showed a significant shrinking of the tumours.

On the strength of Fenyo's work, John Stephenson has set up a medical company headed by Dr Nicol Clark, for polarised treatment in England.

PHOTODYNAMIC THERAPY

At the heat end of the light spectrum, a new treatment using red light, called photodynamic therapy, or PDT, was pioneered in the 1970s by Dr Thomas Dougherty, a research chemist working in New York (see his papers, 'Photoradiation Therapy – new approaches', Seminars in Surgical Oncology 6–16 and 'Photosensitisation of Malignant Tumours' in S. Ecomon, Lea & Febinger, 1980). He found that when porphyrins, light sensitive complex organic compounds forming the basis of respiratory pigments, for example haemoglobin and myoglobin, were injected into the bloodstream, they would be eliminated from all but malignant cells. When the patient was subjected to ultraviolet light, the malignant tumours 'lit up'. Dougherty then found that illuminating these tumours with red light caused them to die.

Since this treatment's crude beginnings, great strides have been made. PDT treatment is now administered with soft laser light and fibre optics. Heading the field in this therapy are the Japanese and Americans. In Britain, research is being carried out by Professor Stanley Brown at the Centre for Photobiology and Photodynamics at Leeds University, where they have recently developed 'interstitial' PDT. This treatment works with large and deep-seated tumours and involves inserting two- or three-fibre optics through which red light is administered into the tumour. This treatment is not yet available to the public. Professor Stanley Brown has also worked with red light around the site where a malignant tumour has been surgically removed to eliminate any cancer cells which still remain.

In summarising this chapter we can see how light and colour has been used in complementary and conventional medicine throughout the ages. Each time it has faded into the background it has been re-discovered and its benefits have become more widely known. With the growing awareness of the detrimental side effects produced by chemical drugs and the effects that invasive surgery has upon both the physical and subtle anatomy, more people are searching for safer and more effective ways to rid themselves of disease.

Many of the ancient seers predicted that as we move into the next millennium the vibrational frequencies of the Earth and all things that live upon it will move into a new level of consciousness and awareness. If this is true, and I believe that it is, will a more refined way of healing be required? If it is, then conventional medicine as we know it will be too crude. If we are beings of light, and this seems to have been verified by auric photography and aura imaging, and we are moving nearer to our true spiritual origin, then treating disease with light and the colours which constitute light seems very right. As the old saying so rightly says, if we are sick, we are 'off colour'. With the latest light research being carried out by people such as Samoilova, Brown and Fenyo, I believe that light will become a great panacea in conventional as well as complementary medicine. Steiner said that light and colour would play an important role in the twenty-first century and Liberman said that light would be the medicine of the future. I also believe this having seen and experienced the power of light and colour when used in healing. But, as I say to my students, don't believe what I say, go and prove this for yourself and at the same time, be open to the light which is present inside as well as outside yourself.

CHAPTER 3

COLOUR

COLOUR COMBINING

Colours originate from light or pigment and their variegated hues and shades are produced by colour combining. Mixing dyes or pigments or superimposing transparent coloured filters is called 'subtractive colour mixing' because the colour obtained is the result of the simultaneous or successive subtraction of various colours from the light passing through the pigment or combination of filters. Mixing light is 'additive mixing' because the resultant colour is the result of combining or adding together colours.

If we mix illuminatory colours, the result will be different from mixing pigment colours. When Isaac Newton experimented with the colours of light he demonstrated that when all the spectral colours are mixed together they produce white light but later experiments have shown that only three of the 'additive' primary colours are needed. These are red, green and blue (blue-violet). These three primary light colours can be used to produce all possible colour sensations. Mixing red and green light produces yellow, green and blue make turquoise or cyan and the combination of blue-violet and red gives magenta. When working with pigment or 'subtractive' colour, white cannot be produced from colour combining but when the exact shades of cyan, yellow and magenta are mixed, black is produced (see page 38). If the exact shades of these colours are not used, the result of mixing them will be a dirty muddy brown.

The number of colours used by colour practitioners varies with each individual practitioner. I personally work with the 12 tertiary colours with the

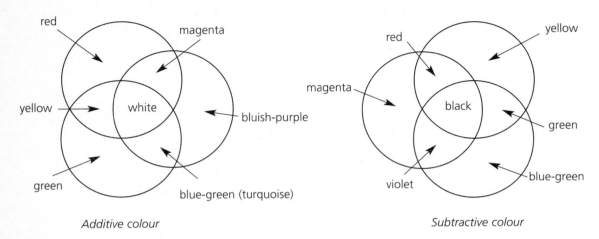

Additive colour   *Subtractive colour*

Mixing colours

addition of rose pink, amethyst, silver and pearl. The tertiary colours are produced by combining the three primary colours to produce the secondary colours orange, green and violet and then mixing each of the secondary colours with its flanking primary colour to produce the tertiary colours red-orange, gold (orange-yellow) lime green, turquoise, indigo and magenta (see Plate section). Adding white to any of these colours will produce a lighter shade and adding black gives a darker shade.

Complementary pairs of pigment colour are those which, when mixed together in the same proportion, produce grey; with coloured light, such a mixture would produce white. A colour's complementary colour is found diagonally opposite it on the tertiary colour wheel; for example, the complementary colour of red is green.

A way of perceiving this phenomenon for yourself is by staring fixedly at a colour until a halo of light starts to appear around its circumference, then transfer your gaze to a white surface and you will see the complementary colour appear as an after image.

CHARACTERISTICS OF THE COLOURS

⚙ RED

Red has the longest wavelengths and lowest energy of all visible light. To focus on a red object, the lens of the eye has to adjust, giving the illusion that the object is closer than it truly is. On the electromagnetic spectrum, red is situated next to infrared, which associates this colour with warmth. In the Victorian era, when heating was restricted to the kitchen, it was customary to wear a red nightshirt to help maintain body temperature and today red gloves or socks are often worn during the winter months.

Red is a 'loud' colour which tends to make it the 'super colour' of the spectrum and its aggressive qualities link it with war and combat and with the masculine energies. The saying 'roll out the red carpet' comes from its link with royalty when a red carpet was laid out for visiting royalty and dignitaries as a mark of respect. This colour has exciting and stimulating qualities, which is why it tends to be used in restaurants to stimulate the appetite and conversation. Red also has the ability to constrict and a room decorated in this colour appears to be smaller than it is. This power of constriction makes red an unsuitable colour for asthmatics.

The names associated with the varying shades of red are derived from the colour's source. Crimson and carmine are taken from the Latin *kermesius*, the name of the dye extracted from the kermes insect. Vermilion is taken from the ancient name for mercuric sulphide, cinnabar, and ruby red, thought to be a very exclusive dye which made it extremely expensive, came from the root of the *Rubia tinctoria* plant.

Physically, red is linked with the heart, blood and flesh and therefore associated with life and love. Ancient man thought that blood held the secret of life and this accredited the colour with special powers. Certain Native American tribes daubed their corpses with red ochre to symbolise their eventual return to earthly life. It is the colour associated with sexuality and with the arousal of sexual energy.

Exposure to red light quickens the heart rate, increases the blood circulation to engender a sense of warmth and prompts the release of adrenaline. Ronald Hunt, in his book *The Seven Keys to Colour Healing* (C. W. Daniel, 1971), states that red splits the ferric salt crystals into iron and salt. The red corpuscles absorb the iron and the salt is eliminated by the kidneys and skin. This makes it a good colour with which to treat iron deficiency and anaemia. This colour's ability to increase circulation also makes it a good colour to use for viral or bacterial infection. Flooding an infected wound with red light will increase the blood supply to the area, enabling the body's white corpuscles to deal more quickly with the bacteria. As already mentioned, red light has been used in America by Dr Thomas Dougherty for the treatment of cancer and this work is at present being researched in England by Professor Stanley Brown.

Red's power to increase circulation, activate the adrenal glands and increase blood circulation makes it unsuitable for people suffering high blood pressure, heart disease, asthma, epilepsy and hypertension.

On an emotional level red is the colour which has the greatest impact. It can cause a person to become aggressive, argumentative and angry. If a person becomes 'red with anger', a dull muddy red appears in their aura. Red is also associated with love. Red roses are frequently given to a loved one.

The negative emotional aspects of this colour are usually associated with the adverse sides of love such as lust. Phrases such as 'red light district' and 'scarlet woman' illustrate this.

When white is added to red it transforms it to rose pink, a softer and more delicate colour associated with the feminine energies and with unconditional love. It is a colour associated with good health and well-being as in the phrase 'in the pink'. On an emotional level, pink is used with the heart chakra on those suffering from 'a broken heart' or from melancholia because it has the power to suffuse this chakra with the vibrational energy needed to overcome the trauma.

☼ ORANGE

Orange is a secondary colour created by mixing together equal portions of red and yellow. It gained its name during the tenth or eleventh century from the Arabic word *nananj*, meaning 'fruit'. It is an earth colour and can be found in the Earth's crust in the form of iron compounds. It is strongly connected to autumn, when the leaves turn the many shades of orange.

The dyes to produce a rich vibrant orange did not appear until the nineteenth century. They were produced by mordanting (or fixing the colour) from a madder, which is a plant with small yellow flowers and a red, fleshy root. The deep, luxurious shades that we find in fabrics today are produced from synthetic dyes.

Orange appears next to red on the colour spectrum. It is a warm colour but does not possess the vibrant heat of red. It is the main colour displayed by the hot spices used in Eastern countries, which verifies its connection with warmth and stimulation.

Like red, this colour is associated with sexuality and fruitfulness. The ancient custom of adorning brides with orange blossom was symbolic of this. Its link with sexuality may stem from the fact that orange is the colour which radiates from the sacral chakra, a chakra which is linked to the female reproductive organs and with the feminine energy. In past eras the orange seeds of the pomegranate were taken as an aphrodisiac.

Orange is the colour of joy and has the power to encourage freedom and movement on all levels of our being. Its vitality is able to bring about a change in our biochemical structure which affords relief from depression. This colour can assist cases of severe rheumatism by helping to break up the deposits laid down in the skeletal structure; it acts as a general tonic; has an antispasmodic effect upon the physical body, making it a favourable colour to use for muscle cramp and spasms; and when applied to the spleen it will give vitality. Furthermore its warm, invigorating nature lends itself as an emotional stimulant.

RED-ORANGE

Red-orange is a combination of equal quantities of red and orange and possesses the qualities of both these colours. It is less aggressive and in treatment, where red is indicated, I have found it preferable to use this colour. Its combination of both the male and female energies creates within it a wholeness and harmony which is transmitted to the patient.

YELLOW

The English word 'yellow' is derived from the Indo-European word *ghelwo*, related to gold. It is the colour nearest to the sunlight and its sunny disposition radiates warmth and inspiration.

Pure spectral yellow occupies a narrow band in the spectrum compared to the other primary colours. Most of the yellow we perceive comes from a mixture of red and green light. Yellow has the highest reflectivity of all the colours and is the characteristic colour of spring because many spring flowers radiate it. In food, especially fruit, it signifies the presence of iron and the vitamins A and C. Spectroscopically, yellow predominates in all herbs which are purgative or nerve stimulants, such as senna.

From medieval times yellow has signified sickness. This relationship may have originated from the yellow pallor afforded to the skin and whites of the eyes in those suffering jaundice. Yellow is the colour of the quarantine flag for ships at sea.

Yellow is a nerve stimulant. It clears the nervous system of stagnant energy when applied to the brow chakra, head and spine. Its positive magnetic currents, which are both stimulating and inspiring, make it a beneficial colour to use with skin problems and for rheumatic and arthritic conditions. It also helps the body to metabolise calcium, which makes it a good colour for those suffering from osteoporosis or calcium deficiencies.

Spectral yellow works with the intellect and with mental inspiration, making it a beneficial colour to use, in small quantities, in studies and places of learning. Being completely surrounded by this colour for a long period of time could cause a state of emotional and mental detachment.

The negative attributes of the colour revolve around cowardice. This link could have arisen from sixteenth-century Spain where people found guilty of heresy and treason were made to wear yellow before being burnt alive.

❀ GOLD

Gold is said to symbolise the universal spirit in its perfect purity. The metal is mined in the United States, South Africa and Canada. Steiner believed that all gold was once part of the sun's ether and the Incas referred to gold as 'the blood of the sun'.

Gold is used extensively in anthroposophic medicine. It improves the circulation and increases body warmth and is said to be a good salve for lupus and skin cancer. In homoeopathy, it is used for depression and suicidal tendencies. In Western medicine gold has long been used for various arthritic and rheumatic conditions, tuberculosis and spinal problems.

This colour is derived from mixing together orange and yellow and therefore contains some of the properties of both these colours. It is a warm and lustrous colour with good light-reflecting qualities. It possesses numerous religious connotations through its association with divinity, with martyrs and the majesty of Christ.

Like yellow, gold applied to the spleen gives vitality to the human system and has a beneficial effect on the skeletal structure of the body, helping to break up the deposits caused by rheumatism and arthritis. Applied down the spine it gives vitality to the nervous system.

☼ GREEN

Green is the colour found midway on the spectrum and it is linked with a sense of balance in all aspects of ourselves. In nature it is the colour of life, found in the new foliage of spring, and decay, seen as mould on rotting vegetation. The eyes focus green light almost exactly on the retina, making it a very restful colour for them. Green's beneficial effects on the eyes has been known since ancient Egyptian times, when green malachite was used as a protective eyeliner. The soothing quality of this colour is why, for more than 300 years, theatres have offered a backstage sanctuary, known as the Green Room, to actors awaiting call or entertaining friends. These benefits could be utilised by those working with computers or for long hours under artificial light by spending their lunch break outdoors among the many shades of green supplied by nature.

Green is the colour of the planet Venus and is therefore associated with love. It was traditionally worn at weddings in Europe, where it symbolised fertility.

This is an unassuming colour and unlike red or red-orange tends to fade into the background, where it does not demand our immediate attention. We can experience this by walking through a forest or through green fields.

The greens of vegetables and herbs are produced by the many kinds of chlorophyll present. Some green leaves are tinged with yellow, due to the presence of yellow carotenoid pigments. If we are successful at growing and caring for both plants and vegetables, we are said to be 'green fingered'.

Being the general colour of nature, green provides nourishment, cools the blood and animates the nerves. As the colour of balance, it is able to bring stability to both mind and emotions and is beneficial for some heart conditions.

The negative qualities associated with green are nausea, poison, envy and jealousy. A person overcome with jealousy is said to look 'green with envy' and one suffering sickness is said to 'look green'. When the body is diseased, it generates unpleasant greens in the form of urine, pus and phlegm.

⊙ LIME GREEN

Lime green is formed by mixing together yellow and green. The main use of this colour in healing is for clearing toxicity caused through a bad diet or chemical substances and for soothing inflammation. This makes it an excellent colour to use on a toxic liver, kidneys or colon. When applied to the throat chakra it cleanses the whole etheric body and the bloodstream. Lime green applied to the brow chakra will cleanse the sinuses of catarrh caused by food allergies or toxicity.

⊙ TURQUOISE

Turquoise is the first colour to appear at the cold end of the spectrum. It consists of blue and green. The proportion of blue to green used determines it as blue turquoise or green turquoise.

Turquoise is the national colour of Persia and the source of some of the oldest and finest turquoise gemstones which they call *piruesh*, meaning 'joy'. Ancient Persians believed that the colour afforded to this gemstone could 'ward off the evil eye', giving protection to their animals as well as to themselves.

As a therapeutic colour, the cooling properties of turquoise work well with inflammatory conditions and help boost the immune system. If the cause of a weak immune system is stress or cigarette smoking, it is advisable to take one gram of vitamin C in conjunction with this colour. Both smoking and stress deplete the body of this vitamin, which is needed to strengthen the immune system.

✿ BLUE

Blue is situated at the cold end of the spectrum. We may be described as being 'blue with cold'. In nature this colour surrounds us in the vast expanse of sky. The sky's colour is produced by sunlight scattering atmospheric particles of the same wavelength as blue wavelengths, causing blue light to be reflected in all directions.

In many of the world-wide religions blue is ascribed to deities. In both the Greek and Roman pantheons it represented their respected gods Zeus and Jupiter. In the Christian religion it is the colour of the mantle worn by the Virgin Mary, signifying that she is Queen of Heaven.

One of the negative attributes of the colour is profanity, as in 'blue film' and 'blue language'. These sayings may have evolved from the expression 'blue gown', the name given to a prostitute, most probably because this was the colour of the dress they were made to wear when entering a 'house of correction'.

On a physical level blue is associated with sadness and depression and from this may have come the saying 'feeling blue'. This makes it an unfavourable colour for those suffering from either of these conditions.

However, blue promotes a sense of peace and relaxation, making it a good colour to have in a bedroom, meditation room or in a room set aside for relaxation. Because of its cold qualities, it is not advisable to use a lot of it in rooms which see very little sun and are potentially dark, but it is good for rooms which benefit from the sun throughout the day.

Unlike red, blue is a colour of expansion and will make small spaces appear larger. For this reason it is a beneficial colour for asthmatics. Other diseases benefiting from this colour are high blood pressure, stress, insomnia and tension. To treat fear and tension, blue should be applied to the solar plexus and for sleeplessness to the brow, throat and solar plexus chakras.

✿ INDIGO

A wonderful description of indigo is 'the vault of heaven on a moonless night'. Its rich, deep colour is obtained by combining equal quantities of blue and violet. Before the introduction of synthetic dyes, this colour was obtained from the indigo plant, but the methods used to produce the natural dye were lengthy and costly, which made it almost unobtainable in the 1940s. It was the jeans revolution in the 1950s that brought back its popularity. Prior to this it was a fashionable colour for millions of Chinese, both for peasants and industrial workers, partly due to the fact that indigo does not show dirt as easily as other colours.

In therapy its healing qualities are those of dignity and high aspiration. Indigo is the dominant colour of the brow chakra, making it a good colour for working with our intuition and enhancing our ability to remember dreams. It is purported to have a powerful effect on mental complaints. Physically, it acts as strong painkiller, and psychologically it is able to clear and clean the psychic currents of the body.

Indigo has the power to create infinite space for us to think, feel or just to be. In some people this could create a sense of solitude and isolation, therefore it is advisable to work carefully with this colour. Belonging to the blue ray, it can also promote depression or intensify it in a person already suffering this complaint.

◉ VIOLET

Violet has the shortest wavelength and the highest energy of all the spectral colours and occurs in a very narrow band next to ultraviolet light.

In the mineral kingdom this colour is found in the amethyst. The word *amethyst* in ancient Greek meant 'not drunk' and in former ages this stone was carried as a protection against becoming drunk on wine. The idea has been proposed that the large amethysts found in ecclesiastical rings were a safeguard against becoming drunk at church banquets. This colour is linked with spirituality and its appearance in a person's aura suggests that they are following a spiritual path.

In the plant kingdom violet is found in the violet flower, whose oil is still used to flavour drinks and candy and as a perfume. In medieval times this oil was used as a sleeping draught and manganese oxide was the pigment used to make violet stained glass. As a dye it was very expensive to produce, which meant that only royalty and the very wealthy could afford to buy it. Its association with royalty could be where its attributes of self-respect and dignity came from.

Violet is a combination of the masculine energies of red and the feminine energies of blue, which gives this colour the ability to balance these two energies in a human person. In *The Luscher Colour Test* (translated and edited by Ian Scott, Pan Books, 1971) Max Luscher states that homosexuals and lesbians show a preference for this colour. This may stem from the need to find and integrate either their feminine or masculine energies. Luscher also believes that emotionally immature and insecure people are drawn to violet.

The healing quality attributed to violet is physical and spiritual strength, engendered by its ability to teach self-love and dignity, so leading an individual to the state of unconditional love.

❂ MAGENTA

Magenta is produced by combining red and violet, the colours which sit at opposite ends of the spectrum. If we look closelt at the spectrum in three-dimensional form it makes a circle and where the red and violet merge magenta is formed. This colour is identified with personal change, which is able to help us rise to the next spiral of life's evolutionary process.

In the thirties this colour was named 'shocking pink', in the fifties 'hot pink' and in the sixties 'kinky pink'. These names proclaim it as a bright, exciting, fun colour, but some people look upon it as sensuous and voluptuous. This could come from its red content.

Magenta dye was first produced by the French, who called it *fuchsine*, after the fuchsia plant. Some time later it was renamed magenta by the Italians after one of their villages near which an especially bloody battle was fought.

On a physical level magenta is the colour used for the treatment of cancer. Both red and violet lie next to the burning rays of infrared and ultraviolet, giving magenta the power to work with this condition.

Psychologically, magenta enables us to let go of old emotional and mental patterns which stand in the way of our spiritual growth. It is the clearing of these that free us to flow with the tide of life.

❂ SILVER

The metal silver is found in the United States, Canada and Mexico. The name comes from an old Anglo-Saxon term of uncertain origin. It is related to the moon and its shiny appearance acts as a mirror, reflecting our own personality and state of being.

Over many years silver has been used in Western medicine for treating burns, as an eyewash, as a substitute for bones and joints and for ear, eye, nose, throat and vaginal inflammations. Silver salts are used for warts.

Silver is a major remedy in anthroposophical medicine and is specifically associated with the female reproductive organs. It is sometimes given to alleviate the pain of childbirth. It aids the brain and circulatory system and acts as a disinfectant. In homoeopathy silver is used for headaches, neuralgic pain in the joints, bronchial congestion and spinal problems.

The colour silver is made from the combination of black and white. This ray has cleansing, burning and cutting qualities and it is used very rarely in colour therapy. Its main use is for cases of obsession, where it is directed at the base of the skull and base of the spine. After application it is vital to seal both these places with the cross within the circle (see page 121). This healing technique should only be practised by those qualified to do so.

○ PEARL

The pearl stone is largely composed of calcium carbonate and is produced by certain molluscs. It is thought that the word 'pearl' is either a translation of the Latin *perla*, meaning 'little pear', or *pilula*, meaning 'a ball'.

The American psychic healer Edgar Cayce said that the pearl activates purity, strengthens the body and stimulates creativity. It is associated with the moon and feminine energy.

When this colour is applied to the solar plexus it is beneficial for abdominal complaints brought on through emotional imbalances and stress, and for feelings of stress and anxiety. When applied to the throat chakra and the spleen it will break up and disperse blockages or serious disharmonies in the etheric body.

A way of helping to clear etheric disharmonies is to solarise water with pearl (see page 173) and add approximately half a glass to your bathwater. An actual pearl can be added to amplify the effect.

CHAPTER 4

THE AURA

EVERY HUMAN BEING is surrounded by an interplay of constantly changing colours, known as the aura. Through techniques such as Kirlian photography this can now be captured on a photograph. The aura is ovoid in shape with the largest part around the head and the smallest around the feet. It is a living part of ourselves that is constantly expanding and contracting with our incoming and outgoing thoughts and feelings. The full extent of its expansion is dependent on a person's spiritual growth and awareness.

The aura is made up of six layers, or sheaths, which interpenetrate each other and the physical body. Each layer has its own vibrational frequency which changes when there is disharmony either in itself or in any of the other layers. The degree to which a person is able to perceive the aura is determined by the range of frequencies they are able to 'tune' into. When the gift of auric sight starts to open, for most people only the layers closest to the physical body are perceived, but with practice and spiritual development this vision expands.

THE ETHERIC BODY

The first layer of the aura, the one closest to the physical body, is the etheric. This is sometimes referred to as the 'etheric double' because it is the subtle counterpart, the energetic blueprint, the light-filled archetype of the physical body. Its energetic magnetism attracts physical matter to produce the coherent physical body as we know it. The etheric framework underlies and permeates every part of the physical body and extends for up to 5cm beyond it. It is the great unifier and when we think of or study this we need to think in non-separative terms.

Alice Bailey talks about the value of the creative imagination and the one great reality it conveys. This is the idea that there is 'no possible separateness in our manifested planetary life – or elsewhere, for that matter'. She says that the concept of separateness, or individual isolation, is an illusion of the unillumined human mind. All forms of life are intimately related to each other through the planetary etheric body (of which all etheric bodies are integral parts). Differences only exist within the levels of consciousness. Alice Bailey concludes, 'There is only one life, pouring through the mass of forms which, in their sum total, constitute our planet as we know it.' (*Esoteric Healing*, 1980; *The Soul; the Quality of Life*, 1974; *A Treatise on White Magic*, 1951 – all published by Lucis Press).

Our etheric body is the vehicle of the soul and is composed of millions of tiny energy channels, called nadis, through which *prana* flows. *Prana* is derived from the sun and is in abundance on a clear sunny day but diminishes in quantity when the sky is overcast. While the nadis appear as separate strands, in reality they consist of one interlocking cord known as the silver cord whose intricate weaving forms the enteric web that surrounds and permeates every form. These nadis are closely linked with the nervous system in the physical body. Where the cords of this energetic strand pass over each other, energy centres or 'chakras' are formed. The size and potency of the chakra depends upon the number of energy lines involved. Where seven cross an acupuncture point is formed, 14 create a minor chakra and 21 a major chakra. Each of the major chakras is linked with one of the physical body's endocrine glands.

The functions of the etheric body not only make our carnate life possible through its assimilation and transmission of *prana* but also allow us to contact, experience and register that which we perceive as 'outside' ourselves through working with our five senses. These provide access to the tangible world for the soul. Without these functions we would truly be alone.

The etheric body is controlled by thought, therefore to bring it into its full functioning and glorious state needs right, elevated and pure thinking.

When working with the etheric body in relation to healing it is important to remember that the etheric itself is never sick. What it does do is to absorb both internal and external conditions, which ultimately manifest as physical disease if not dealt with. The internal conditions arise from our emotional and mental states, and the external conditions, which cause the etheric body to become devitalised, are environmental pollution, the lack of vitality in chemically produced and genetically engineered food, food additives and microwave cooking.

It is thought by many esoterocists that etheric congestion has become a major cause of difficulty for the masses of humanity due to age-long habits of suppression and inhibition, both of which prevent the full functioning of the chakras and inhibit the flow of *prana*. I believe that we have reached a point in the history of mankind when we truly have to look at ourselves in order to eradicate all old thought patterns and genetic traits which we no longer resonate to. It is the act of doing this that frees us from the illusion we call life and leads us to discover our true divine selves and fulfil our potential as human beings.

Other difficulties experienced by the etheric body can be due to the connection between the dense physical form and the etheric counterpart being too loose. This produces a devitalised and debilitated condition, making the individual susceptible to ill health. It also means that the soul cannot fully integrate with its vehicle. Mild forms of this condition produce a tendency to faint. Extreme forms include obsession and possession. If, on the other hand, the etheric body is too tightly integrated with the physical body, disorders of the nervous system can arise.

Something that still remains a mystery is the effect of physical surgery on the etheric body and nervous system. It has been suggested that the flow of *prana* through the nadis is short-circuited due to its loss of contact with that specific part of the physical body and therefore there is no need to supply the removed organ with vitality. One avenue of thought is that new bridging channels of force are established within the etheric body, but how this occurs and what adjustments are made are still unknown.

THE MAJOR CHAKRAS

The word 'chakra' is derived from Sanskrit and means 'a wheel' or 'circle'. The seven major chakras are formed in the etheric body but interact with the rest of the aura and the physical body. Five of these chakras are situated in line with the spine and the other two lie between the eyebrows and just above the crown of the head. These chakras are powerhouses of energy which work with the physical body to energise and activate it. Each chakra radiates one of the spectral colours and is connected to one of the endocrine glands in the physical body. On a higher level they form a spiritual ladder leading to enlightenment. In therapy these are very important centres to work with, especially with individuals suffering hormonal problems.

In Indian philosophy the major chakras are symbolised as lotus flowers, each bearing a specific number of petals. These petals are inscribed with Sanskrit letters and at the centre of each flower various animals, gods and goddesses reside, each ascribed with symbolism.

The Base Chakra

The Sanskrit name given to this chakra is *Muladhara, mula* meaning 'root' and *adhara* meaning 'base' or 'support'. The chakra is situated at the base of the spine and is usually depicted with four petals radiating its dominant colour, red. It is associated with the element earth and the sense of smell. It influences the blood, spine, nervous system, vagina, legs and bones. The endocrine glands associated with it are the testes.

This chakra is the seat of the kundalini or serpent fire. The esoteric spine, which is the blueprint for the physical spine, houses a thread composed of three strands of energy. These three strands are known as the *pingala*, *ida* and *sushumna*. The *pingala* is the positive strand which channels the dynamic energy of *prana*. It is associated with the sympathetic nervous system which releases adrenaline to stimulate the superficial muscles. The *ida* is the negative strand, relating to the path of consciousness and psychic unfoldment. It is connected with the parasympathetic nervous system which sends impulses to the visceral organs to stimulate the internal process. The third thread is the *sushumna* and is the path of pure spirit, providing a channel for the great human spiritual energy force. These three paths channel electric fire, solar fire and fire by friction. The kundalini fire is the union of these three fires and only when a person has reached a certain stage in their spiritual development can this energy be raised rapidly and safely.

The base chakra has a very close connection with the physical body, providing it with vitality and strength. It is connected to our instinct of survival and procreation and is responsible for integrating us with the Earth. Its polarity is the incoming and outgoing breath. To transcend this chakra is to work at rising above animal survival instincts.

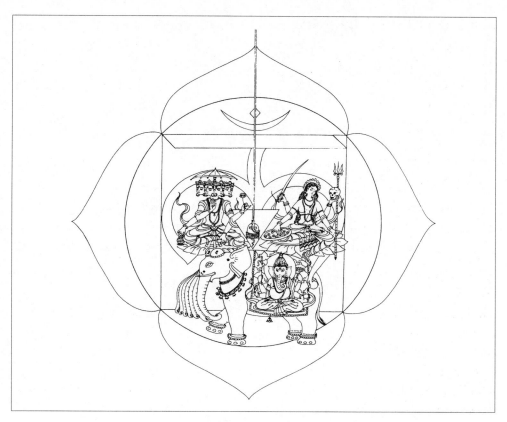

The base chakra

When this chakra's energy is balanced it provides vitality and brings a sense of well-being to the physical body, leaving a person grounded and cen-tred, sexually affectionate and the master of themselves. Excessive energy can lead to aggressiveness, make a person domineering, egoistic and sexually aggressive. Deficient energy creates a lack of confidence and depression accompanied by little will-power to achieve one's aims in life. It makes a per-son uninterested in sex and invariably they are not grounded.

Some of the physical symptoms that could manifest when this chakra is not functioning to its full potential are spinal and leg problems, testicular dis-orders, inhibited rejuvenation of blood cells and haemorrhoids.

The Sacral Chakra

In Sanskrit the name for this chakra is *Svadistana*, meaning 'abode of the vital force'. It is situated just below the navel and is shown with six petals radiating its dominant colour orange. It is connected to the element water and the sense of taste. It works with the female reproductive organs, the mammary glands, the skin and the kidneys, and its associated endocrine glands are the adrenals.

This is a very powerful centre, controlling a person's sex life and thereby linking with creativity, especially in the female. This chakra also has a close link with the creative energies at the throat chakra, which displays its complementary colour, blue. When a woman is passing through the menopause, the creative energies from the sacral chakra are transmuted to the throat chakra, where they are transformed into spiritual energies. Unfortunately, anyone taking hormone replacement therapy stops this transformation.

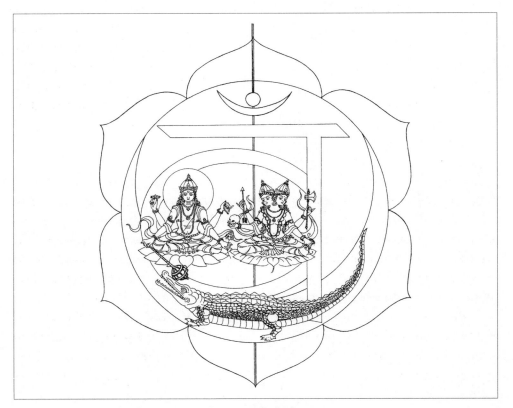

The sacral chakra

The sacral chakra is the source of vitality for the etheric body. It influences our feelings of sexuality and governs our love/hate relationships. Its polarity is of attraction and repulsion, likes and dislikes, feelings which govern our desires. To transcend this chakra is to rise above our likes and dislikes and to see all things as part of the whole.

When this chakra is balanced, a person shows concern for other people, is friendly, optimistic and has a sense of belonging. Their sexual energy is balanced and they are attuned to their own feelings. When functioning to its full potential, this chakra opens a person's intuitive powers and heightens their sensitivity. If the chakra becomes overcharged, a person can become emotionally explosive, aggressive, overly ambitious, manipulative, overindulgent and obsessed with sex. If it becomes blocked and deficient in energy, a person could become oversensitive, extremely shy and fearful, resentful, distrustful and burdened by guilt. Sexually they could be frigid or impotent and a female could experience difficulty conceiving.

The physical symptoms which can arise from the malfunctioning of this chakra are bladder and kidney disorders, circulatory problems, intestinal complaints, shallow and irregular breathing accompanied by frequent low energy, disturbances of the central nervous system, migraines and irritability. Dysfunction in either the male or female reproductive organs can also result. In the male this could show as impotency and in the female it could result in the inability to reach orgasm, in infertility or in menstrual disorders.

The Solar Plexus Chakra

The Sanskrit name given to this centre is *Manipura*, which means 'the jewel of the navel'. It is situated just above the navel and is symbolised by 10 petals radiating its dominant colour yellow. It is associated with the element fire and the sense of taste. The parts of the body influenced by it are the skin, digestive organs, stomach, duodenum, pancreas, gall bladder and liver. The associated endocrine glands are the islets of Langerhans which form part of the pancreas. This chakra is the fire wheel and is associated with the sun and with the ego. It is the centre of digestion known to the Chinese as the 'triple warmer' because heat is generated in the process of digestion. Its polarity is power and powerlessness and when we are able to transcend this polarity the result is peace.

This chakra is linked with the emotional or astral body and as well as

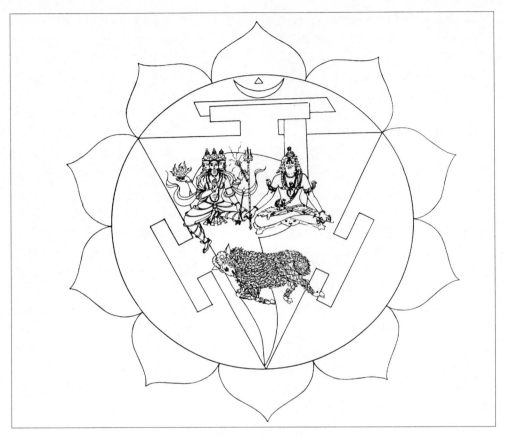

The solar plexus chakra

responding to our feelings it reacts to thoughts of worry, anxiety and fear. It is a centre of extreme importance in the life of the average person because humanity is conditioned by desire and this is the centre through which most of these energies flow. It is important for those people who are psychic or sensitive to make sure that this centre is protected because it is where the thoughts and emotions of other people can be picked up and where energy can be consciously or unconsciously withdrawn by individuals who are lacking strength and vitality.

When the solar plexus chakra is balanced in energy, a person has self-respect and respect for others, and is outgoing, cheerful, relaxed, spontaneous and uninhibited. They enjoy physical activity, good food and show emotional warmth. Excessive energy in this chakra can make one judgemental, a workaholic, a perfectionist and resentful of authority. If the chakra is depleted of energy it can lead to a state of depression, confusion and insecurity. The person may lack confidence and worry what other people think of them. They could be afraid to be alone and also suffer from poor digestion.

Some of the physical symptoms that can arise from an imbalance in this chakra are stiffness, muscular and nervous tension, stomach and digestive problems, problems with the lower back, diabetes, hypoglycaemia, liver problems, low vitality and fevers.

The Heart Chakra

The Sanskrit name for this chakra is *Anahata*, which means 'the unstruck or unbeaten sound'. It is situated near the fifth thoracic vertebra and is depicted with 12 petals which radiate its dominant colour, green. It is identified

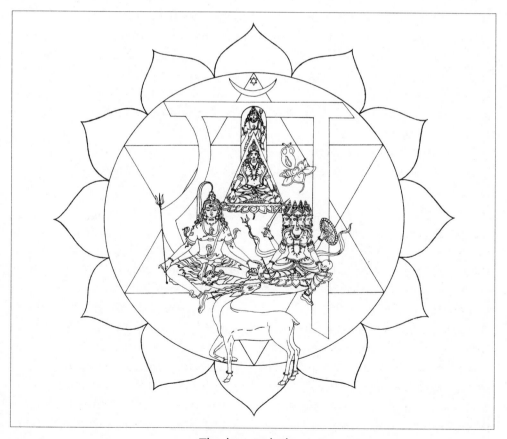

The heart chakra

with the element of air and the sense of touch. It influences the heart, lungs, the immune and circulatory systems and lymph glands. The endocrine gland with which it is associated is the thymus. It is linked to the mental body, which makes its polarity thought coming in and thought going out. When we are able to transcend this polarity, we transcend mind to connect with divine love.

This is the centre where we experience love. *How* we experience this depends upon how open and evolved this centre is. Love can be felt at a purely physical level, either as sexual arousal or lust, or it can be transformed into the unconditional love which encompasses all things. Before reaching this state we have first to love all aspects of ourselves. As we achieve this, our love is slowly transformed into the unconditional love which is able to reach out to all beings and all conditions we encounter, without judgement.

When this chakra's energies are in a state of balance it generates compassion, a desire to nurture others and a growth towards unconditional love. A person feels balanced, and compassionate, is friendly, outgoing and in touch with their feelings. If this centre has excessive energy it can make a person demanding, over-critical, possessive, moody, depressed and a master of conditional love. Deficient energy can create paranoia, indecisiveness, a desire to hang on to objects or people, a fear of rejection and of being hurt and a need for constant reassurance.

When this chakra is malfunctioning the physical symptoms which can arise are breathing problems, lung diseases, asthma, high blood pressure and heart disease.

The Throat Chakra

In Sanskrit this centre is known as *Visshudha*, which means 'to purify'. It is located at the first cervical vertebra and is shown as a blue 16-petalled lotus. It is related to the element of ether and to the sense of hearing. On a physical level it works with the throat, ears, shoulders, the parathyroids and the thyroid gland. It is also linked with the digestive tract, through the oesophagus, with the genital organs, through the thyroid gland, with the lungs and bronchial tubes, and is closely connected with the centre of speech.

This chakra is connected to the higher mental body and is one of the most important centres in healing. Treating it affects the whole of the etheric body through the nervous system, in much the same way as the spleen affects the

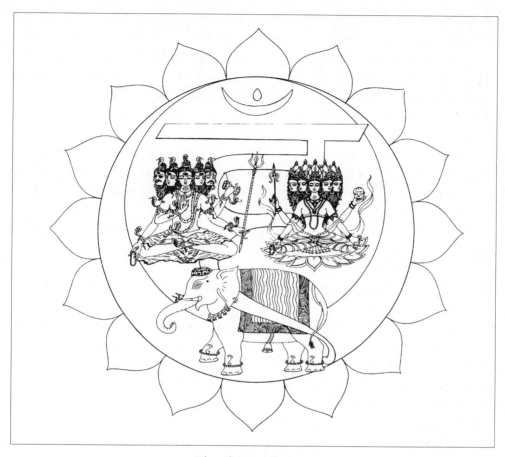

The throat chakra

whole of the physical body through the intake of life force. The throat chakra is connected to creative intelligence and to the spoken word. It registers the creative purposes of the soul, transmitted to it by the inflow of energy from the brow centre. The fusion of these two energies leads to creative activity. This chakra's polarity is life and death. To transcend life and death is to know the immortal or spiritual self, yet still as an individualised conscious being.

Near to the back of the throat and connected to the throat chakra lies the lalana gland. When this is stimulated by higher yogic practices it produces a sweet nectar which is claimed can sustain a yogi for any length of time without food or water.

Balanced energy here makes a person contented, centred and a good speaker. They can be musically or artistically inspired and are able to meditate and experience divine energy. They have no difficulty living in the present and have an easy grasp of spiritual teachings. If this chakra is over-stimulated it can make a person arrogant, self-righteous, dogmatic and an excessive talker. They may also possess excessive sexual energy. If it is deficient in energy, it can make a person scared, timid, inconsistent, unreliable, devious, manipulative and afraid of sex.

Some of the physical symptoms which could arise from a malfunctioning throat chakra are exhaustion, digestive and weight problems, thyroid problems, sore throats and throat infections, neck pain and pain in the back of the head.

The Brow Chakra

This chakra is located on the forehead, midway between the eyebrows. The Sanskrit name given to it is *Ajna*, meaning 'to know' or 'to command'. It is usually depicted with two indigo petals which speak of the duality of human nature, the yin and the yang and the masculine and feminine energies which are inherent in all human beings. This chakra also reflects the twofold nature of the mind, the ego self and the spirit self, the reasoning and the intuitive mind. When this centre is open and functioning to its full potential the duality is integrated into wholeness and the energy resident here is raised to the crown chakra and to God consciousness. It is closely related to the causal body.

On a physical level this chakra is related to the brain, eyes, ears, nose and nervous system. Its associated endocrine gland is the pituitary, whose secretions influence all the other endocrine glands. When treating this chakra and the crown chakra we are contacting the highest aspects of a person's soul, therefore our highest aspects should be employed in this service.

When this chakra is balanced and functioning to its full potential we are unattached to material possessions, have no fear of death and are not preoccupied with fame or fortune or worldly things. The inherent gifts of telepathy and astral travel open and we are able to access past lives. Our veil of illusion is pierced and we recognise ourselves as a tiny part of the whole of creation.

If this chakra is vibrating with excess energy, we can become proud, manipulative, religiously dogmatic and an egomaniac. Too little energy can

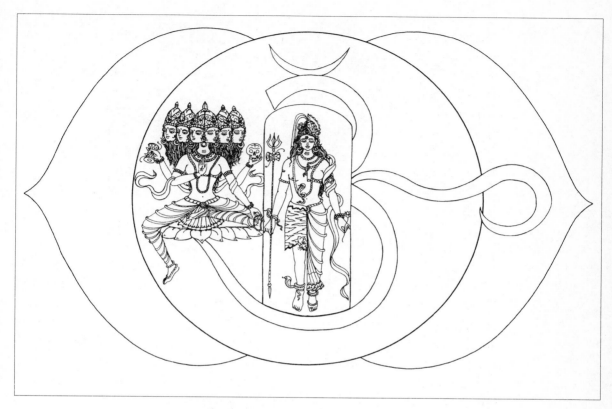

The brow chakra

make us oversensitive to the feelings of others, afraid of success, non-assertive, undisciplined and unable to distinguish between the ego self and the higher self.

Some of the physical symptoms which may arise when this chakra is out of balance are headaches, eye problems, sinus problems, catarrh, hayfever, sleeplessness, migraine and hormonal imbalances.

The Crown Chakra

This centre's Sanskrit name is *Sahasrara*, which means 'thousandfold'. It is located just above the crown of the head and is symbolised by a thousand-petalled lotus radiating violet. In the physical body it governs the nervous system, the brain and the pineal gland.

At this centre we have reached the top rung of the ladder. Our lower and

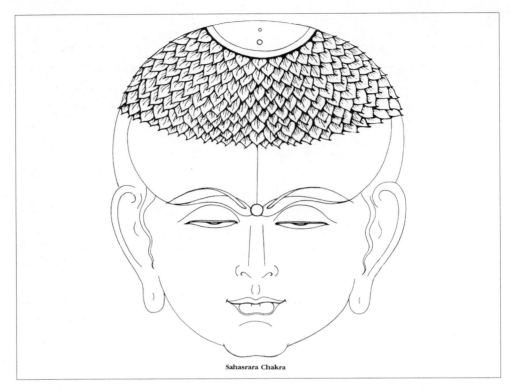

Sahasrara Chakra

The crown centre

higher selves have been united, enabling us to experience the indescribable bliss of union with the divine reality found in each one of us. When this complete illumination takes place, the brow and crown chakra unite to form the halo depicted in the pictures of saints and enlightened beings.

When this chakra is open and functioning to its full potential we become open to divine energy. This enables us to transcend the laws of nature and have total access to the unconscious and subconscious mind. Too much energy here can cause a constant sense of frustration and frequent migraines. Too little energy and we are indecisive and lack that vital spark of joy.

The physical symptoms which can arise from the malfunction of this chakra are brain disease, migraines, disorders of the endocrine system and psychological problems.

The Alta Major Chakra

This chakra is situated at the medulla oblongata. It radiates the colour magenta and governs the carotid glands. These are small reddish-brown structures situated one on each side of the neck where the carotid artery divides. Their main function is controlling breathing to maintain an adequate supply of oxygen to the tissues of the body. Oxygen levels are maintained by a reflex operating between the carotid gland and the respiratory centre in the brain.

Triangles of Light

The three chakras situated in the head with their respective glands and the right and left eye form three triangles of light at a set stage of a person's spiritual development (see below).

Two of these triangles are distributors of energy and one is a distributor of force. When these triangles are linked up, they produce a magnetic, radiant field which enables a healer to project colour or healing force from the brow chakra (see page 64).

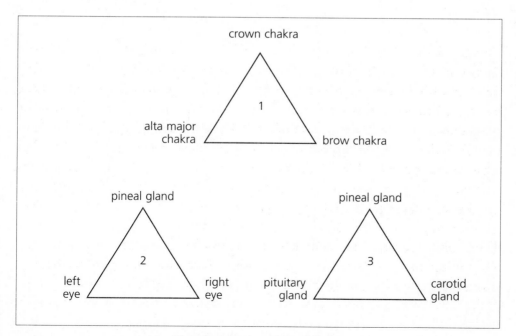

The three triangles of light

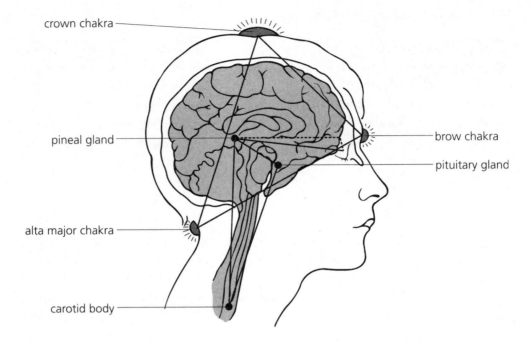

crown chakra

pineal gland

brow chakra

pituitary gland

alta major chakra

carotid body

The linked triangles

The alta major chakra is employed in raising the kundalini energy. Cosmic energy pouring down through the crown chakra to the brow chakra combines personality and soul energy. Then, by an act of will, this combined energy is projected down the spinal column via the alta major chakra to the base chakra where it combines with this chakra's energies. When this happens, the union of the three fires takes place and the kundalini energy rises with great force to bring enlightenment.

THE MINOR CHAKRAS

The 21 minor chakras are connected to organs throughout the physical body and radiate to a subtle shade of the major chakra located nearest to them. It is important to work with these chakras in healing especially if the nearby major chakra's associated organ is suffering from disease. Table 1 shows where these chakras are situated and their associated colour.

The two spleenic chakras are of great importance. It is here that vitality

Table 1: The Minor Chakras

Position of minor chakra	Associated colour
One behind each eye	A shade of indigo
One at the base of each ear	A shade of indigo
One midway along each clavicle	A shade of blue
One in the palm of each hand	A shade of blue
One near the thymus gland	Turquoise
One near the nipple of each breast	A shade of green
One near the liver	A shade of yellow
One connected to the stomach	A shade of yellow
One connected with the gonads (female ovaries)	A shade of orange
(male testes)	A pale shade of red
One behind each knee	A shade of red
One on the sole of each foot	A shade of red
Two connected with the spleen	Orange/gold

from the sunlight is absorbed and distributed throughout the etheric body via the seven major chakras. If a person suffers from a weak and anaemic physical body these two minor chakras should always be treated with either orange or gold to promote physical strength and vitality.

THE ASTRAL OR EMOTIONAL BODY

This layer of the aura interpenetrates with both the physical and etheric bodies but because it is slightly larger it extends beyond them for up to 30cm. The astral body is an aggregate of forces which manifest as feelings, wishes, desires, longings and aspirations. Its glory lies in the fact that it can literally reproduce any form which we desire. An example of this is astral projection. If our emotional intention is to project our astral body to a desired place, a body-like form will appear there. This is the power of the astral world.

The astral body is able to assume any shape or form it desires and is truly a master of disguise. It can be likened to the image of water. If you look at an object in water it will always appear distorted through water's ability to bend light. If the water is calm and still the distortion of the object will be minimal, but if the water is turbulent the object will be barely discernible. If sediment is churned up by the water's turbulence, our perception of the object will be further clouded. The same principle applies to the astral body. Depending upon the orientation of an individual, their astral body will either respond to the churning world of the senses, which will lead to continual mood swings and emotional upsets, or to the stabilising influence of the soul. The latter can only occur when we have learnt to become the master of this aspect of ourselves.

An interesting aspect of the astral body is its disappearance as we reach the state of perfection and enlightenment. Great spiritual teachers like the Buddha and the Christ are purported to have had no astral emanation. Their auras were purely spiritual and because they were no longer limited by the restriction of personality attachments they were able to extend their aura over a vast radius.

One of the principal features of the astral body are the colours which constantly flow through it. These are an expression of our feelings and emotions. All known and at present unknown colours are displayed throughout the layers of the aura. As we move towards the outermost layer, the colours become more subtle and ethereal. Below are listed the colours most frequently found in the astral body together with their related emotion.

RED   Deep red flashes, usually against a black background, symbolise anger.
A cloud of scarlet shows irritability.
A dull and heavy crimson denotes selfish love.
Brilliant scarlet against a light background denotes 'noble indignation'.
Pure, clear red is physical love.

ROSE PINK This colour shows unselfish love. When joined by violet it becomes linked with unselfish love for humanity.

ORANGE   A clear orange is joy and optimism.
A dull, muddy orange shows pride or ambition.

YELLOW   A clear bright yellow relates to intellectuality.
A dull yellow is linked with selfishness.
Primrose yellow is linked with an intellect that is devoted to spiritual pursuits.

GOLD	This shows an intellect that is pursuing philosophy or the wisdom of sacred geometry.
GREEN	A dull muddy green points out envy. Green lit up by deep red or scarlet flashes shows jealousy.
BLUE	A clear blue expresses spiritual devotion.
BROWN-GREY	This dull hard colour is related to selfishness.
BROWN-RED	This colour is usually perceived as parallel bars across the astral body and is connected with avarice.
GREY	A heavy dull grey shows depression. A very bright, livid grey is linked with fear.
BLACK	Black, seen as thick clouds, shows hatred and malice.

An interesting concept to consider is the 'care and feeding' of the astral body. The astral body does slowly wear away and therefore needs replenishing. To do this, instead of eating and digesting food like the physical body, it attracts replacement particles from the surrounding astral environment. Just like the physical body, the astral body's health depends upon the quality of 'particles' attracted. A good astral diet comes from constructive feelings, uplifting aspirations and selfless love.

The astral body has three general functions. These are: to make sensation possible; to serve as a bridge between the mind and physical body; and to act as an independent vehicle of consciousness and action. One of its most destructive forces is fear, but one of its most potent forces is joy, which can heal and cleanse the physical body. Foster Bailey in *Reflections* (Lucis Press, 1979) shows how valuable joy is to both healer and patient.

In this book, he explains that joy is much more than a pleasant sensation, 'It is a precipitation of an aspect of the life of the human soul into the life of the personality and a combining with it.' Joy has specific energies which can be detected and developed. It helps to heal and protect because it harmonises and creates a positive condition. Joy is a force which is acceptable to everybody, arouses no resentment and kills jealousy. It produces self-assurance and poise. Bailey says thinking about joy helps it to develop within ourselves and recognising its value opens the door to acquiring it. 'True joy is quiet and evidences an inner peace.'

THE MENTAL BODY

The mental body is larger in size than the astral body and is composed of more refined matter. Its development comes from constructive, active thought and not from idle conversation or from passively watching television. The amount of thought determines its growth and the quality of thought determines the kind of matter employed to achieve that growth.

The mental body is said to be an object of great beauty. The delicacy and rapid motion of its particles give it an aspect of living iridescent light. Its beauty becomes more radiant as the intellect becomes more highly evolved and more consistently orientated towards spiritual concepts. Every thought creates a vibration in the mental body which is accompanied by a play of vivid, delicate colour.

The mental body rotates rapidly on its axis, creating a series of bands throughout its structure. These bands are not always clearly defined nor always uniform in width, but they are distinguishable to those with clairvoyant sight and in approximately the same position in each individual. Each band has a spiritual colour which vibrates to one of the 49 shades associated with that colour and is determined by the thought process of the individual.

Aspirational thought is usually seen as a small violet circle at the top of the mental body. As a person's spiritual aspirations grow, the circle increases in size and radiance. In the initiate it manifests as a glowing cap of vibrant violet. Below this lies the narrow blue ring of devotional thought followed by a much broader band relating to affectionate thought. Depending on the type of affection, the colour displayed in this band can be any shade of crimson or rose pink. Near to this layer and often connected to it is an orange band, an expression of proud and ambitious thought. Intimately related to this is a yellow band which manifests from philosophical and scientific thought. The location of this yellow zone varies in different people. Sometimes it fills the whole of the upper part of the mental body, rising above affection and devotion. If a person is very proud, it becomes excessive.

Every thought that we think creates a shape or form and the broad belt devoted to these occupies the middle section of the mental body. The principal colour here is green, mixed with shades of yellow and brown. This is the most active part of the mental body, crowded with a continuous, ever-changing stream of thought forms. These forms can be projected into the atmosphere, to places and to people through visualisation. Like attracts like, therefore if we harbour negative thoughts, these will attract other negative thoughts of a like nature, thereby amplifying the negativity. If we think positively, these thoughts will be augmented in the same way. This knowledge should teach us to be conscious of what we are thinking and to change any negativity into positivity.

If an initiate passes into the mental world and communicates there with another being, their communication is through colour, sound and form. This conveys the complete thought as a colourful, musical picture instead of the mere fragment that is shown on the physical plane by the symbols we call words. This form of communication is called telepathy and whether or not we are aware of it, we are constantly surrounded by, immersed in and subject to telepathic interplay.

Clearly, thought plays a major role in healing. Indeed, healing is a thought-directed process. One of the seed thoughts of the Maitreya School of Healing is: 'The healer recognises life as flowing processes and supports the patient within the movement of their individual process.' It is the capacities of the mental body that make the healing processes possible.

THE HIGHER MENTAL BODY

The higher mental body lies next to the mental body and extends beyond it. Its size is dependent on the development of the intuition. As colour practitioners, the development of this layer of our aura is of prime importance. There are set colours for specific diseases, but each person is an individual and this sometimes necessitates the use of a different treatment colour from the norm. The only way of discovering this colour is by listening to our intuition. Dowsing, or working with a pendulum, is another way in which we can work with the intuition (see pages 78–9). Again, to work efficiently and correctly with this we must employ trust. Initially this can prove difficult because it is not easy to immediately discern between the imagination and the intuition, but with practice and trust this faculty will develop.

The colours which flow through this part of the aura are dependent upon how open our intuition is and to what extent we are influenced by the mental body. In an evolved person pale shades of blue and violet permeate throughout.

THE CAUSAL BODY

This layer is so named because it is where the cause for our present incarnation is stored. When we choose to reincarnate we do so with certain tasks to perform and situations to experience. These aid our spiritual growth and development. Unfortunately, from the time of our birth we are conditioned, which causes us to lose sight of our purpose. However, if we have learnt to listen to and trust our intuition, this will guide us to and along our chosen path in life.

This layer of the aura houses information on all past lives but unless it is necessary for our growth the average person is unable to access these. I feel that we have enough to cope with in this lifetime without trying to relive the traumas of past lives.

In most people this layer and the next layer of the aura are not yet fully developed, making the colours which are displayed there difficult to see by the few people who have the ability to see these layers of the aura.

THE BODYLESS BODY

This body represents our true self, our divinity which has no beginning and no ending. It is the essence which knows all things and which has chosen to incarnate into a physical body in order to experience certain conditions only in existence on the Earth plane. The most important of these conditions is that of free will, the liberty to choose our way in life. Working with the other layers of the aura leads us to the glory and divinity of this one – a practice which takes many lifetimes to accomplish.

CHAPTER 5

THE USE OF COLOUR IN THERAPY

L EARNING ABOUT THE aura teaches us that we are beings of light, surrounded and interpenetrated by the colours which constitute light. So we need natural daylight as part of our daily diet. Sunlight contains the *prana* needed to feed our etheric body, which in turn is responsible for revitalising our physical body. *Prana* constitutes the spectral colours which are utilised by the chakras to feed the endocrine glands and to revitalise and harmonise all the other layers that make up our subtle anatomy.

The easiest way to absorb light is through the eyes and to absorb *prana* is through the breath. This can be achieved by spending a minimum of 30 minutes each day outdoors without spectacles or contact lenses. The lenses of some spectacles and contact lenses are made from glass or a plastic which does not allow ultraviolet light to pass through, therefore these should be removed for the duration of time you spend outdoors. To absorb the maximum amount of *prana*, be conscious of your breathing whenever you spend time in the open. Try to use the full capacity of your lungs and make your inhalation the same length as your exhalation.

FEELING 'OFF COLOUR'

When we become unwell, we are literally 'off colour'. Parts of our aura either vibrate to the wrong colour frequency or are devoid of colour. In the majority of people this imbalance stems from the emotional body which registers our feelings and stress levels. If the cause of this imbalance is not found and rectified, it will eventually be reflected as a physical disease.

The work of a colour practitioner is to help the patient find and work with the cause of the disease they present with and to keep them in a state of homoeostasis while they work with themselves. For many people the idea of working with themselves is a new concept and could necessitate many changes in their lives which may initially create a state of distress and insecurity. Part of the healing process is the challenge to work with these changes because they provide us with wonderful opportunities for growth at all levels of our being. Unfortunately a large percentage of the population has been conditioned to rely upon their doctors to maintain their health and if they do become ill, they feel that their only responsibility in recovering is in remembering to 'take the tablets three times a day'. This is a false concept. I believe that our bodies are self-healing given the right conditions and if we do become sick there is a cause which we need to work with. Having said this, I do believe that allopathic medicine has its place. There are some conditions which need medical intervention, but I also believe that these conditions are learning curves and the only way to learn from them is to take a long, hard look at ourselves.

We have learnt that our emotional and mental bodies interact with the physical, and traumas experienced at this level will be reflected physically. I look upon the physical body as a mirror which reflects all that is happening at the subtle levels of our self. It can also succumb to disease through outside influences such as pollution and devitalised food. These produce stagnated energy into the etheric body, preventing the free flow of *prana*, or the food itself may be so depleted of *prana* that we ourselves become depleted.

This can be helped through the appropriate use of colour.

COLOUR THERAPY TECHNIQUES

In therapy, there are many techniques for using colour. The method I employ utilises colour in three ways. These are through what I term the *general colours,* the *treatment colours* and the *overall colour.*

General Colours

These are the colours to which specific parts of the physical body naturally vibrate to and are, with a few exceptions, determined by the dominant colour of the nearest major chakra. In contact healing these colours are used to revitalise and balance the organs of the physical body and to clear any associated stagnant energy accumulated in the etheric body. The general colours attributed to the physical body are shown in Table 2.

Table 2: **The General Colours**

Body part	General colour	Complementary colour
Pineal gland (Crown chakra)	Violet	Yellow
Pituitary gland (Brow chakra)	Indigo	Gold
Eyes	Indigo	Gold
Ears	Indigo	Gold
Sinuses	Indigo	Gold
Neck	Blue	Orange
Thyroid gland	Blue	Orange
Parathyroids	Yellow	Violet
Shoulders	Blue	Orange
Arms	Blue	Orange
Hands	Blue	Orange
Lungs	Green	Red
Heart	Green	Red
Breast	Green	Red
Kidneys	Yellow	Violet
Adrenal glands	Yellow	Violet
Liver	Yellow	Violet
Gall bladder	Yellow	Violet
Stomach	Yellow	Violet
Pancreas	Yellow	Violet
Spleen	Orange/yellow	Indigo
Small intestine	Orange	Blue
Colon	Orange	Blue
Bladder	Orange	Blue
Ovaries	Orange	Blue
Fallopian tubes	Orange	Blue
Uterus	Orange	Blue
Prostate gland	Orange	Blue
Testes	Turquoise	Red-orange

continues

Body part	General colour	Complementary colour
Legs	Red	Green
Feet	Red	Green
Skeletal system	Yellow	Violet
Immune system	Turquoise	Red-orange
Circulatory system	Violet	Yellow
Nervous system	Gold	Indigo
Spinal column	Yellow	Violet

The Treatment Colour

This is the colour administered either with light or through contact healing to work with a physically manifested disease. The colours given in Table 3 are the ones which are used for most people, but there is a small percentage who may need to be treated with a different colour. You can find this out by listening to your intuition or by dowsing (see pages 78–80). It is very important to remember that with each of these colours its complementary colour must be used.

The diseases listed are the ones more commonly seen in complementary practice. To list the vast number of diseases which afflict man would require writing a very large dictionary!

Table 3: **The Treatment Colours**

Body part	Complaint	Colour	Complementary colour
Spine	Paralysis	Yellow	Violet
	Injury or pain	Indigo	Gold
Head	Epilepsy	Blue	Orange
	Headaches	Indigo	Gold
	Migraine	Indigo	Gold
	Neuralgic pain	Indigo	Gold
	Insomnia	Indigo	Gold
	Head colds	Orange	Blue
	Amnesia	Violet	Yellow
	Alzheimer's disease	Yellow	Violet

continues

Body part	Complaint	Colour	Complementary colour
Pituitary gland	Tumours	Magenta	Lime green
Sinuses	Sinus pain	Indigo	Gold
	Infection	Red-orange	Turquoise
Neck	Stiff neck	Blue	Orange
	Sore throat	Red-orange	Turquoise
	Laryngitis	Red-orange	Turquoise
Eyes	Eye strain	Indigo	Gold
	Cataracts	Indigo	Gold
	Infection	Red-orange	Turquoise
Ears	Tinnitus	Magenta	Lime green
	Ear infection	Red-orange	Turquoise
	Ruptured eardrum	Indigo	Gold
	Ménières disease	Orange	Blue
Thyroid gland	Simple goitre	Blue	Orange
	Overactive thyroid	Blue	Orange
	Underactive thyroid	Orange	Blue
Parathyroids	Osteoporosis	Yellow	Violet
Shoulders	Muscular strains and tension	Indigo	Gold
	Arthritis	Yellow	Violet
	Frozen shoulder	Indigo	Gold
Breast	Cysts	Magenta	Lime green
	Cancer	Magenta	Lime green
	Mastitis	Blue	Orange
Lungs	Asthma	Blue	Orange
	Bronchitis	Orange	Blue
	Cancer	Magenta	Lime green
	Pneumonia	Turquoise	Red-orange
Heart	Tachycardia	Blue	Orange
	Palpitations	Blue	Orange
	Thrombosis	Magenta	Lime green
	Angina pain	Indigo	Gold
	Broken heart (emotional)	Violet	Rose pink
Solar plexus	Tension and stress	Blue	Orange

continues

Body part	Complaint	Colour	Complementary colour
Gall bladder	Gallstones	Orange	Blue
Liver	Toxicity	Lime green	Magenta
	Jaundice	Blue	Orange
	Cirrhosis	Violet	Yellow
Stomach	Indigestion	Yellow	Violet
	Ulcers	Blue	Orange
	Cancer	Magenta	Lime green
Pancreas	Diabetes	Yellow	Violet
Spleen	Low immune system	Turquoise	Red-orange
	Enlarged spleen	Magenta	Lime green
	Low vitality	Gold	Indigo
Kidneys	Nephritis	Turquoise	Red-orange
	Kidney stones	Orange	Blue
	Nephroma	Magenta	Lime green
	Water retention	Magenta	Lime green
Bladder	Cystitis	Red-orange	Turquoise
	Cancer	Magenta	Spring green
Small intestine	Inflammation	Indigo	Gold
	Cancer	Magenta	Spring green
	Crohn's disease	Indigo	Gold
Colon	Constipation	Red	Green
	Diarrhoea	Blue	Orange
	Diverticulitis	Red-orange	Turquoise
	Cancer	Magenta	Spring green
Ovaries	Ovarian cyst	Orange	Blue
	Pregnancy	Blue	Orange
	Infertility	Red	Green
Uterus	Pregnancy	Blue	Orange
	Cancer	Magenta	Lime green
	Fibroids	Orange	Blue
	Infertility	Red	Green
Lymphatic system	General treatment	Turquoise	Red-orange
	Lymphoma	Magenta	Spring green

continues

Body part	Complaint	Colour	Complementary colour
Joints	Arthritis	Yellow	Violet
	Inflammation/pain	Indigo	Gold
Prostate	Enlarged	Blue	Orange
	Cancer	Magenta	Lime green
Testes	Cancer	Magenta	Lime green
	Infertility	Red	Green
Anus	Piles	Yellow	Violet
	Inflammation	Indigo	Gold
Skin	General problems	Violet	Yellow

THE OVERALL COLOUR

This is the colour which helps a person find and work with the cause of the physically manifested disease. I have given it this name because it works with and is administered to the whole person and because of the work it does. I feel that it is the most important colour.

The overall colour is usually administered, with its complementary colour, as light through the colour therapy instrument (see pages 171–3). For this it is important that the patient is dressed in white, otherwise the colour they receive will be a combination of the colour administered and the colours of the clothes they are wearing.

In situations where it is not possible to work in this way, the colour can be given for a shorter duration of time through the soles of both feet because the feet are a mirror image of the person, the microcosm of the macrocosm. The method used for this technique is visualisation (see pages 175–7). At the end of the general treatment, place both hands on the soles of the patient's feet and visualise first the overall colour being channelled through your hands and into the feet, followed by the complementary colour. Each colour should be visualised for approximately two to three minutes.

There are three ways of finding the overall colour needed to treat someone. The first is through dowsing, the second through kinesiology and the third through the spinal diagnostic chart (see next chapter).

Dowsing

It is thought that dowsing originated from the tools used by shamans when entering into communication with the spirits. When difficulties were experienced the shaman would use a stick, originated from the magician's wand, or a pebble hung on a thread to direct questions at. The direction in which it moved answered yes or no to his question. A variety of similar devices have been used for divination ever since. The best known is the forked hazel twig commonly used to dowse for water, oil and missing objects.

In the 1920s a French priest, Abbé Mermet, claimed to have used the ancient art of water divining or dowsing as a means of locating and diagnosing illness. He gave demonstrations of his skill in hospitals to which, as a member of a religious order, he had access. The doctors at the hospitals selected groups of patients for him to work with and with the aid of his pendulum he would diagnose their ailments. The accuracy of his diagnosis frequently surprised onlookers and mortified sceptics. On the strength of his discoveries he wrote *Principles and Practice of Radiesthesia* (London, 1975), a term used to describe dowsing for medical purposes.

Dowsing works on the principle that all substances, including the physical body, emit radiation. If a person is able to 'tune in' to this radiation their body acts as a receiver for some intangible current flowing through their hands. When dowsing for water or oil, the divining stick or pendulum indicates the location of these substances by picking up their radiation and the strength of their radiation. The greater the strength, the more substance present.

If you choose to work with a pendulum it is important to possess your own. This should be cleansed from any old or negative vibrations prior to your using it. The simplest way of doing this is to leave it in salt water overnight and wash it the following morning under running water. When you have cleansed it, carry it around in your pocket for a couple of weeks to enable it to become permeated with your own vibrational energy.

Learning to work with a pendulum takes time and patience and requires you to work with and trust your intuition. The first step is to discover your 'yes' and 'no' response. To do this, hold the pendulum approximately 15cm away from your solar plexus and mentally ask it to indicate your 'yes'. It will respond by swinging either clockwise or anti-clockwise or in a horizontal or diagonal line. Now ask it to indicate your 'no'. Again it will respond in the same way. Once established, these responses should always be the same for you.

When dowsing to glean information on a patient, something that holds their vibration is needed. In the past a spot of blood was used but this is no longer necessary or safe with the risks involved from HIV and hepatitis. Instead, a photograph of the patient, a piece of their hair or their handwriting can be used. The object is placed beneath the pendulum when dowsing.

Initially, dowsing can produce doubts in our mind and we may wonder if the information we have collected is correct. The lesson we need to learn from this is trust.

Dowsing Exercise

An exercise which is good for practising your dowsing skills is to place under a group of white mugs or cups a piece of different coloured paper or a different object. Then shuffle the mugs or cups around so that you do not know which colour you have placed under which mug. Then, with your pendulum, try to discover which colour or object is beneath each of the mugs or cups. If you only get one or two right, don't be disheartened, practice makes perfect. When your skills start to improve, ask a friend or a member of your family to hide an object somewhere in your home and see if you can find it with the aid of your pendulum.

Dowsing for the Overall Colour

To do this you will need to make yourself a small disc, approximately 8cm in diameter, containing the eight overall colours (see page 80). This you place on your patient's hand. Then ask your pendulum to indicate the overall colour needed by them. Your pendulum will swing diagonally across two colours, maybe blue and orange, for instance. You then ask your pendulum if blue is the overall colour. If it indicates 'yes', blue will be the overall colour with orange as its complementary colour. If it indicates 'no', the colours are reversed, with orange as the overall colour and blue its complementary.

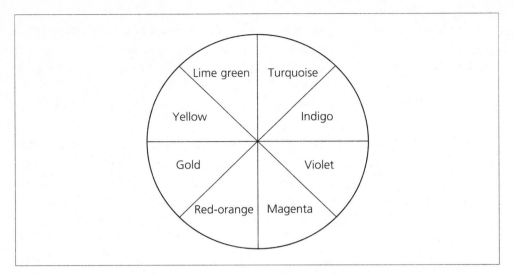

The colour wheel for dowsing the overall colour

Kinesiology

Kinesiology is the study of body movement. It was introduced by Dr George Goodheart, a chiropractor from Detroit. Combining Eastern ideas on energy flow with his own chiropractic techniques, Goodheart developed a system that used muscle testing to determine the effectiveness and need for treatment. He then used various kinesiology techniques to restore muscle balance. (For further information see A. Holdwatt, *Kinesiology*, Element Books, 1995.)

Practitioners working with kinesiology do not diagnose illness but look for imbalances or deficiencies in nutrition and energy and diagnose food allergies. The body is thought to recognise and react to nutrients and chemicals and these reactions affect the way muscles work. If a substance placed on the tongue causes instant muscle weakness, this indicates that the person is allergic to the substance.

Finding the Overall Colour with Kinesiology

To work with this method you will need 12 coloured cotton swatches or 12 pieces of stained glass.

First test the muscle tone of your patient by using your fingers to gently press down on their outstretched arm. Repeat this, asking your patient to resist your pressure. Having ascertained their muscle tone and resistance, face them towards the light and gently tie in turn each of the eight swatches relating to the overall colours gently around their open eyes. Then use kinesiology with each of the eight colours to find the ones needed by the patient.

If there is more than one colour needed, dowse these to find the overall colour.

If you prefer, squares of stained glass can be used in place of the cotton swatches. These are held by the patient, approximately 5cm away from either their left or right eye. The eye being used remains open and the other eye is closed.

Before using dowsing and kinesiology with your patients, first practise with your friends and family. This will help you to become proficient at these arts and to gain confidence.

CHAPTER 6

※

THE SPINE CHART

A VERY USEFUL AID in diagnosis is the spine chart originated
approximately 20 years ago by Hygeia Studios in Gloucestershire and
developed by the Oracle School of Colour. It is used to find the overall colour
needed by a patient, as an aid to counselling, to determine the state of the
chakras and as a guide to possible energy imbalances in the physical body.

This chart comprises the spine, the skull, 40 small boxes alongside the
skull and spine, and the seven major chakras with the inclusion of the alta
major chakra. The musical octaves down the side of the chart are the work
of Olivea Dewhurst Maddock, author of *The Book of Sound Therapy* (Gaia
Books, 1993) and the initiator of integrating sound with reflexology (see
Plate section).

The human spine comprises 33 vertebrae divided into 7 cervical, 12 thoracic, 5 lumbar, 5 sacral and 4 coccyx. The four coccygeal vertebrae are fused
into two bones. Enclosed in the bony vertebral column is the spinal cord.
This is a soft column of nerve tissue continuous with the lower part of the
brain. Except for the 12 pairs of cranial nerves which connect directly with
the brain, all the spinal nerves of the body enter or leave the spinal cord
through openings between the vertebrae. All the functions of the body
depend upon the integrity of this intricate mass of cord tissue. The brain and
the spinal cord are jointly known as the central nervous system. The brain is
encapsulated in the skull which is constructed from eight flat bones.

On the spine chart the fourth coccygeal vertebrae is where the base chakra
is situated. The remaining 32 vertebrae are divided into four sections of
eight vertebrae. The first section of eight vertebrae, encompassing the coccyx,

represents the physical body, the next section portrays the metabolic process, the third section stands for the emotional body and the fourth section the mental body. The eight flat bones of the skull, symbolised on the chart as eight small boxes inside the skull, represent the spiritual aspect. Each of these five sections contains the colours red-orange, gold, yellow, lime green, turquoise, indigo, violet and magenta. The seven major chakras situated alongside the skull and spine radiate to their dominant colours of red, orange, yellow, green, blue, indigo and violet, and the alta major chakra glows with magenta (see Plate section).

CONSTRUCTING A CHART FOR A PATIENT

Dowsing the Chart

To make a spine chart dowsing is used. The patient's signature is marked along the spinal column on the back of the chart as a witness or if preferred, their photograph can be placed beneath the chart.

When dowsing the chart always start at the head and work down to the base of the spine, as this allows for the higher healing energies to be brought down through the head to all other aspects of the person. It is never a good idea to work in the reverse order for fear of raising a person's energy, which may not be beneficial for them at that precise moment.

The aim of dowsing is to discover which of the flat bones and which of the vertebrae are vibrating to the wrong energy and the extent of their imbalance. These usually number between 10 and 20. Using a pendulum to do this can be time-consuming, therefore students learn to dowse using their middle finger. This finger is used because it extends the furthest of all the fingers and is the most receptive to outside energies. Working with this method takes practice. The first step is to discover how your finger reacts to energy imbalances. Some general reactions are a prickling feeling in the finger, the sensation of heat or cold or sometimes pain. Once you have determined your reaction, it should not change. When this way of dowsing has been mastered, it is both quick and efficient, but there may be those who still prefer to use an ordinary pendulum and for them this is right.

When making a chart, first ask that you may be an instrument for the higher energies to flow through you for the good of the person you are working with, then, holding the middle finger of either your left or right hand marginally above the first small box in the skull, slowly run your finger down the boxes followed by the 32 vertebrae. Where you feel a reaction in your finger, mark the appropriate boxes or vertebrae with a cross (X). If the reaction that you get is strong, place a plus sign beside the cross (+), if you feel a medium reaction place a circle (O) and if weak use a minus sign (-).

When you have finished dowsing the chart, colour the marked boxes and vertebrae with their appropriate colour (these are given by the side of each box and vertebra), then in the box opposite, enter the complementary colour.

Your first attempts at using this form of dowsing with a chart will necessitate you running your finger over the chart several times to learn your reaction but as you gain confidence it is important that you only dowse the chart once. To continuously go back over it for confirmation leads to confusion and if you are working with your intuition this should not be necessary.

Bridging the Colours

The next stage in the construction of a spine chart, referred to as 'bridging the colours', shows which problems the person is working with and which they are not. These bridges, alongside any unbridged vertebrae, are recorded in the grid found at the bottom of the chart. The letters alongside this grid, starting from the top, stand for spiritual, mental, emotional, metabolic and physical.

To construct a bridge, start with the first colour appearing at the top of the chart. Now look to find the same colour in the boxes housing the complementary colours. If there are more than one of this colour, use the one which is furthest away. For example, if the first colour is magenta in the spiritual and in the complementary boxes this colour appears in both the emotional and the physical, the magenta in the physical would be the one used to form the bridge because this allows energy to be brought through the mental, emotional and metabolic aspects of the person, helping them to work with their problem on all of these levels. A line is then drawn to connect these two magentas.

Because in colour therapy the complementary colour is nearly always used with the treatment colour, the lime green in the complementary box opposite the spiritual magenta is now bridged to the lime green opposite the magenta in the physical by drawing a second line. These two lines form one bridge.

Once a colour or complementary colour has been used in the formation of a bridge, it cannot be used again.

To record this bridge in the grid, draw an arrow from the spiritual section to the physical. The rest of the colours on the chart are then treated in the same way. Any colours that cannot be bridged because they do not have a counterpart in the complementary column are termed 'unbridged' and identified with an asterisk inside a circle. These are also recorded in the appropriate section of the grid (see Plate section).

When the bridging has been completed, the overall colour is found from the unbridged colours. If, for example, two magentas, one lime green, and one indigo remain unbridged, the overall colour would be magenta because this colour is in excess of the others. If there is one magenta, one red-orange and one gold unbridged, the colour with the strongest vibration, detected from the plus, nought or minus signs by its side, is used. If all the colours are the same strength, then dowsing is used to verify the overall colour.

Dowsing the Chakras

When this part of the chart has been completed, the chakras are dowsed with a pendulum to ascertain their state of balance. Those that are in balance are ignored. Those which are overactive are treated during the therapy session with their complementary colour and those which are underactive are treated with their dominant colour. For reference, the overactive chakras can be marked on the chart with a plus sign and coloured with their complementary colour and the underactive chakras can be marked with a minus sign and coloured with their dominant colour.

Because the energy surrounding a person is constantly changing, a spine chart should be made for them either on the morning of their treatment or when they are present. For this reason, a chart made one or two days prior to treatment could be inaccurate. Learning to make and read these charts proficiently requires practice and this is best gained by attending a course where this method is taught.

INTERPRETING THE SPINE CHART

The colours appearing on the chart symbolise the problems facing a patient. If the colour is bridged it shows that they are already working with the problem, if unbridged it indicates that as yet the problem is not being dealt with.

When a chart is analysed the basic structure of the chart is explained to the patient and an interpretation of the colours which appear on it are given. Working in this way encourages a person to open up and talk about their problems as well as giving the therapist insight into the person. If the patient is not familiar with their subtle anatomy, the chakras are not discussed but are treated.

Interpretation of the Spinal Colours

The Spiritual Aspect

RED-ORANGE The appearance of this colour in the spiritual area could be indicative of someone who has not integrated their spirituality with their physical life. These two aspects of ourselves have to be embodied for our greater good. The presence of orange in this colour could point to dogma which is being upheld by the person but which no longer holds any truth for them. This can lead to frustration and apathy instead of uplifting feelings and joy.

GOLD Gold is the colour of wisdom, truth and knowledge, and its presence on the chart shows that a person is not yet versed in the spiritual wisdom which comes from the search for and finding of their divine self. This search requires self-discipline, the practice of meditation and the acquisition of esoteric wisdom gained from following a spiritual path. When spiritual wisdom has been found and becomes part of the person's life it imbues them with everlasting bliss and joy.

YELLOW Yellow is the colour of the intellectual mind and when this colour appears in the spiritual part of the spine chart it indicates that the person has difficulties accepting the aspects of spirituality which cannot as yet be proven. Intellectuals often have difficulty with spiritual teachings because they are constantly trying to prove them. They also have problems listening to and trusting their intuition for the same reason. Their challenge is to learn to trust and to accept that not all spiritual concepts can be proven with the rational mind.

LIME GREEN This colour presents a two-fold challenge. Its presence on this aspect of the chart dares the person to look at any religious dogma present in their life in order to evaluate its effectiveness and worth. Dogma can be likened to putting on blinkers which prevent us from seeing the many ways which lead to divine truth. At some point in our life any dogma which fails to inspire or hold truth for us has to be dropped to make way for new ideas and practices that further our spiritual growth. When a certain point in our spiritual growth has been reached, dogma fails to exist, because we are able to see the truth in all things.

The second challenge that this colour presents is the challenge to integrate what we believe into all aspects of our lives. Some people who are working with meditation, for example, practise this at a set time each day. Krishnamurti, an Eastern sage, wrote that meditation is not a separate thing from life but the very essence of life, the very essence of daily living, and only when the whole of our life has become a meditation have we truly integrated our spirituality into every part of ourselves.

TURQUOISE In the spiritual area this colour could denote a religious fanatic, one who believes that theirs is the only true religious path. The green present in turquoise shows the imbalance of this notion and the blue shows the need to find the unconditional peace and tranquillity necessary in order to understand that all paths ultimately lead to God.

INDIGO This is the colour which portrays the vastness and the silence of space. As above, so below; as without, so within; and spiritually indigo is challenging the person to look for this space and silence within themselves because only when this has been found will they discover their true self. The majority of the population look for security, peace, fulfilment and joy through earthly things, but these are only transient, passing away as quickly as they are found. When we find joy, peace and fulfilment within ourselves these become part of us and therefore can only be destroyed by us.

VIOLET This colour is challenging the person to acknowledge and then start to work with unconditional love. This is the highest form of love and embraces all things for what they are. It never judges or criticises, but understands that whatever a person does is a learning curve for their growth and understanding. When we eventually reach the point where we *become* unconditional love, we never think about it because we *are* it.

MAGENTA When this colour appears in the spiritual aspect of the chart it is indicating the need for greater spiritual awareness in order to make the changes necessary for further spiritual growth. Life is frequently portrayed as a spiral along which we transcend and evolve. In magenta the physical colour of red and the spiritual colour of violet have united to form the magenta of transcendence through change.

The Mental Aspect

RED-ORANGE When red-orange appears here it is indicating a lack of mental energy and joy. This could result from intellectual hard work, in which case the colour would disappear on a chart made after a good night's sleep. Other reasons for its presence are mental worry or boredom. The latter could apply to a woman who has chosen to leave a mentally stimulating career to raise a family.

GOLD In the mental area this colour is indicating a person's inability to listen to and trust their intuition. They believe that all knowledge and insight is gained through their intellect. Any problem-solving or decision-making becomes a pure intellectual exercise. As yet the person does not possess the insight to know that all true knowledge comes from the intuition and that intellectual knowledge is based on someone else's theories – which may not always be correct.

YELLOW Yellow is related to the mind and when it appears in this aspect of the spine chart it is indicating that the person is ruled by their mind instead of being its master. In most people the mind spends every second of every hour producing thoughts on every conceivable topic, an activity which prevents the person from being still to listen to the voice of intuition. Those practising meditation know how difficult it is to quieten the mind and tran-

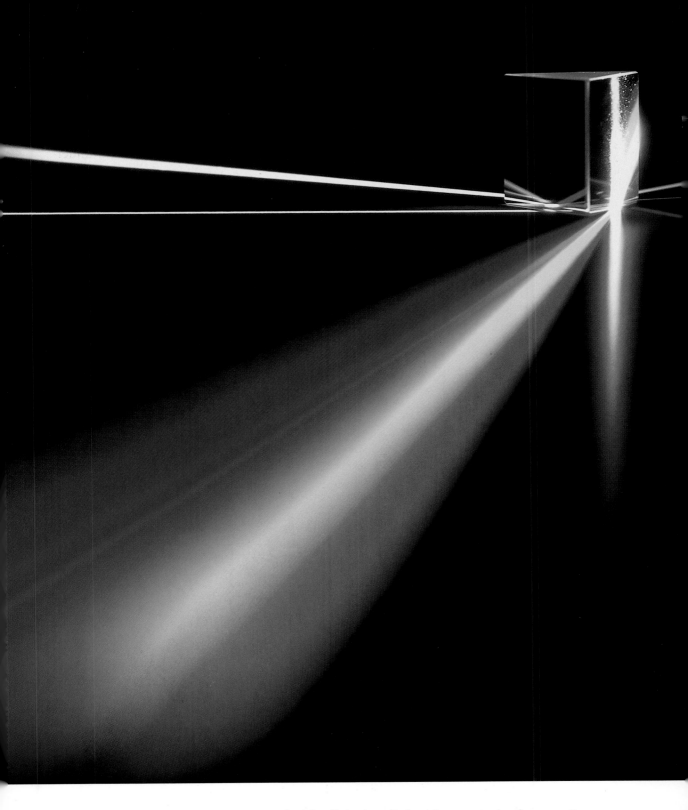

The light spectrum: a beam of white light is split into its spectral colours as it passes through a glass prism.

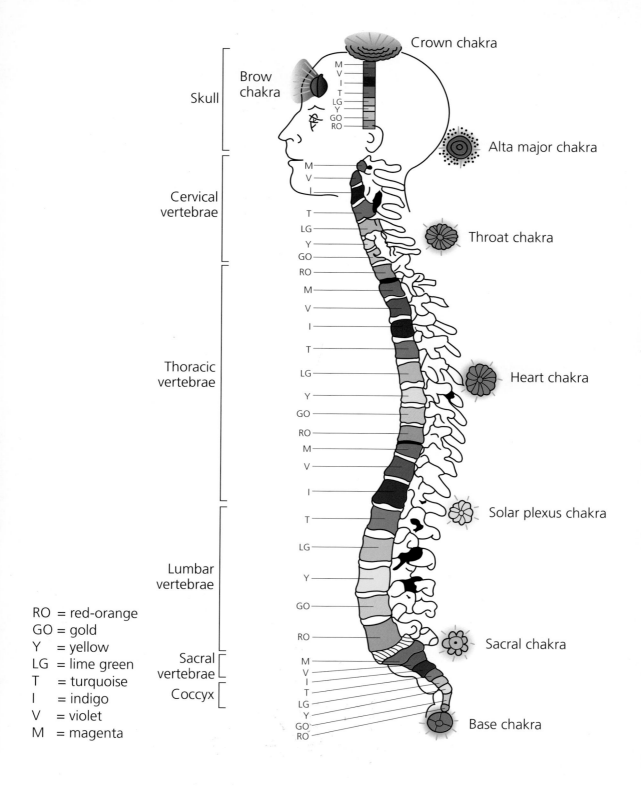

The spine chart showing the colours of the spinal vertebrae.

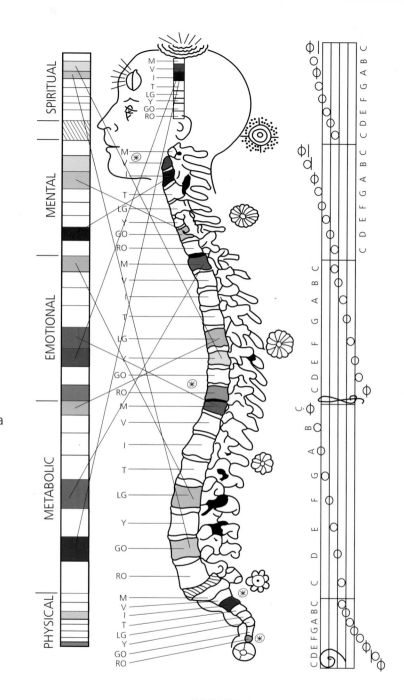

Base chakra = red
Sacral chakra = orange
Solar plexus chakra = yellow
Heart chakra = green
Throat chakra = blue
Alta major chakra = magenta
Brow chakra = indigo
Crown chakra = violet

RO = red-orange
GO = gold
Y = yellow
LG = lime green
T = turquoise
I = indigo
V = violet
M = magenta

SPIRITUAL

MENTAL

EMOTIONAL

METABOLIC

PHYSICAL

Name of patient _____ MRS A _____

Date of chart _____ 10 · 8 · 99 _____

Overall colour required _____ Red-orange _____

SUMMARY GRID

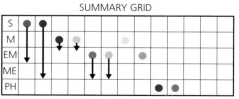

A completed spine chart.

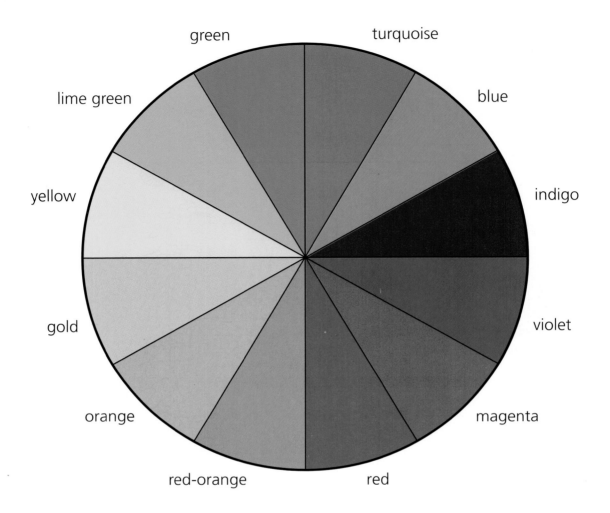

red	= energy (masculine)	green	= balance
red-orange	= joyful/energy (feminine)	turquoise	= immunity
orange	= joy and laughter	blue	= peace
gold	= wisdom	indigo	= space – analgesic
yellow	= stand back	violet	= dignity and love
lime green	= detoxification	magenta	= change

The twelve colour wheel.

scend it into the higher states of consciousness. The lesson this colour teaches is awareness of the mind's activity and the need to explore ways of becoming its master.

Another cause for this colour's appearance in the mental aspect of the chart is mental turmoil. The causes for this are many and to promote a cure the cause must first be found. If there is more than one solution to the problem, it helps to write on a piece of paper all the fors and againsts for all the possible solutions. This exercise frequently provides the answer.

LIME GREEN This colour can portray someone who is very negative in their attitudes or one who is mentally reliving the past. It is showing the need to change this negativity into a more positive attitude to life. For the person living in the past it is useful to look at their past and integrate all its positive events into the present, then lay down what remains to make room for new growth. This can be likened to pruning a tree and removing all the dead wood to enable the tree's growth to be healthier and stronger.

This colour could also be suggesting that there is some degree of mental imbalance. This could take the form of a mental illness or be connected to the left and right hemispheres of the brain. The left hemisphere works with our intellectual pursuits and the right hemisphere with our creativity, both of which should be worked with equally. If our career is intellectually orientated, we need to find a creative hobby and vice versa.

TURQUOISE This colour shows an overactive mind that is impossible to escape from. The presence of blue in this colour shows it is necessary to bring stillness and peace of mind and the green helps to restore its balance. It is important to remember that the mind affects the body in the same way as the body affects the mind. If the mind is in a constant state of agitation it will produce a similar state in the physical body; likewise a quiet and tranquil mind will create a quiet and peaceful body.

INDIGO When this colour appears it portrays mental fatigue and the need to find space for relaxation and rest. This space can be found through a creative hobby, by listening to music or by doing something that gives joy and happiness. The space could be needed for the person to sit quietly and review where their life is taking them and whether or not this is the way they wish to go. If not, they need to consider what changes are needed.

VIOLET On a mental level violet is asking a person to love their thoughts, even the negative ones, and to accept them as part of themselves. Thoughts that are suppressed because of their unsavoury nature will eventually manifest as a physical disease. It is therefore important to face these and talk about them with either a trusted friend or therapist in order to find a way to gently disperse them. Loving yourself can be very difficult for those who have been brought up in a strict religious faith which teaches that this is a selfish thing to do. Unfortunately, if we cannot love ourselves we cannot deeply love anyone else. But when we start to explore love and accept our thoughts for what they are, a harmonious change takes place, bringing with it a greater sense of well-being.

MAGENTA Magenta in the mental area of the chart indicates the need to release old thought patterns blocking the mental layer of the aura. These prevent a person from evolving by obstructing new ideas and experiences. It is very easy to live in the past but what needs to be remembered is that the past has gone and all we need to take from it are the lessons learnt and insights gained. The future may never come. This leaves us with the now, the present. It is this which we are being challenged to work with and live in.

The Emotional Aspect

RED-ORANGE In the emotional area this colour is showing the person to be emotionally drained of energy. The cause of this is usually trauma in their life. Their challenge is to examine the cause of the trauma in order to find a solution. Their lack of emotional energy may also be because they are being drained of it by another individual. If this is happening it is important for them to learn how to protect themselves and take mastery over their own energies (see pages 119–24). The orange contained in this colour speaks of their need for more emotional joy, a lack of which can cause emotional lethargy.

GOLD When gold appears it can be an indication that emotional manipulation is taking place. As yet the person has either not acquired the wisdom which enables them to see what is happening or is taking the easy way out by turning a blind eye to the situation. If this is not wisely and promptly dealt with it can take over a person's life and will ultimately lead to a state of severe depression and hopelessness. Someone who works with emotional manipulation will not easily give up, especially if they are achieving their aims. It is the victim who has to find the strength to resist by walking away.

YELLOW This colour portrays a highly emotional person, someone who is ruled by their feelings and has very little control over them. In such a person the emotional layer of their aura vibrates to the wrong frequency and their solar plexus chakra lacks balance. This could have an adverse effect upon the pancreas, spleen, liver and stomach, either individually or collectively. One of the challenges of our present age is to grow in emotional strength until this part of our aura dissolves, freeing us from the limitations of personal attachments.

LIME GREEN Lime green in the emotional area shows a need for emotional detoxification. It is very easy for the astral body to become blocked with feelings of fear, anger, jealousy and hatred. The only purpose these fulfil is to make us physically sick. Fear will surround a person in a heavy, grey mist which no light can penetrate. It often helps to do the thing that we are afraid of; if angry, work at forgiving by looking at our own shortcomings; if jealous, look at all the blessings which we have bestowed upon us, and if full of hatred, turn that emotion to feelings of love.

TURQUOISE Turquoise is the colour of immunity and its appearance in the emotional aspect of the chart shows that the person is ruled by their emotions. The blue which helps to make up this colour speaks of the emotional peace and tranquillity needed before looking for ways to reverse this situation. The green present helps to stabilise the emotional body. This colour can appear when the person is suffering from a persecution complex or from paranoia.

INDIGO Indigo is the great painkiller and speaks here of the need for the person to look at and resolve their emotional pain. This can be very difficult for them to do and also requires a lot of understanding and patience on the part of the therapist who needs to be a good listener, as well as a good counsellor. Indigo also has the ability to create the space needed for the person to look at and work through their emotional trauma. With time and understanding they will pass through this phase and continue their life with greater wisdom and positiveness.

VIOLET Emotionally violet teaches us to love our feelings and to accept them as part of ourselves. Unfortunately some religious disciplines teach that certain feelings are sinful and will lead to hell and damnation. All that this kind of teaching achieves is to make a person suppress their feelings and become burdened with emotional guilt. Whatever our feelings or desires, we have to look at what they are, and if they are in any way negative or destructive, resolve to change them through love.

MAGENTA This is the colour that shows the need for change in a person's emotional outlook. It requires us to look at old emotional patterns and to eradicate those which no longer serve a purpose. This will bring emotional strength and give us mastery over our feelings. I know from experience that when we start to work in this way, we are tried and tested sometimes to the point where we feel like giving up, but when this happens it is important to remember that all these tests serve to help us achieve our objectives in life.

The Metabolic Aspect

RED-ORANGE The metabolic part of the spine chart deals with how we metabolise the food we eat. When red-orange appears it indicates that we are not absorbing through the small and large intestine all the nutrients from the food we eat. The cause could be intestinal disease, diarrhoea, taking laxatives or stress, which undermines all of our body's systems. Because this colour comprises red and orange, it could be a sign that the person is suffering from anorexia or bulimia. There is no joy in eating. Both of these eating disorders stem from a deep psychological cause and require professional help.

GOLD How often do we eat food purely for our sense of taste and not because we are hungry? When gold appears it is informing the person of the need for wisdom in selecting the foods needed for their optimal health, not for the gratification of their tastebuds. To do this one needs to be in tune with one's body and listen to its requirements. Gold frequently appears on the chart of those who have no time to eat properly, either because they are too tired or too busy or because they cannot be bothered to prepare a nutritious meal. In order to stay healthy and maintain our vitality, we need to eat food which is free from pesticides but full of vitamins and minerals.

YELLOW Yellow is the colour nearest to sunshine and its appearance in the metabolic area of the spine indicates that the individual is lacking calcium. This colour frequently appears on the charts of menopausal women, especially if they spend little time outdoors in natural daylight. It has been proven that ultraviolet light absorbed through the eyes aids vitamin D production, which is needed for calcium metabolism. Yellow is the colour of detachment, so its appearance might also indicate an eating disorder (the person has detached themselves from food) which could have its origins in an emotional or psychological disturbance.

LIME GREEN This colour is informing the person that their physical body is toxic through an unbalanced diet. Toxicity can arise from eating junk food, from food allergies or from constipation. All of these causes have to be looked at if the condition is to be righted. If a therapist feels that their patient's diet is unbalanced or they are suffering food allergies it is always advisable to suggest that they make an appointment with a qualified nutritionist.

TURQUOISE Turquoise is the colour of immunity and its appearance in the metabolic area of the chart indicates that the person is suffering a weak immune system. This occurs in people who are HIV positive or who have recently undergone a viral or bacterial infection. The immune system can also become depleted through stress or smoking cigarettes. Both of these sap the body of vitamin C, which is vital for the maintenance of our immune system, therefore a vitamin C supplement would be beneficial for these people.

INDIGO When indigo appears metabolically it suggests that the person's digestive system is under stress from either an emotional or mental problem. I am sure that many of you have experienced a curbing of your appetite when passing through a stressful or emotional situation. This is nature's way of protecting the body by not allowing the stomach to be filled with food which at that moment cannot easily be digested. Alternatively, this colour provides space and needing digestive space typifies the person who never stops eating. Food represents comfort, mother, love, and if these are lacking in a person's life they may be trying to fill the void with food. This condition requires a lot of counselling alongside treatment.

VIOLET If we are to gain the maximum benefit from the food we eat we need to take time to prepare nutritious food, allow ourselves sufficient time to eat and digest it and to bless the food prior to eating it. Blessing our food heightens its vibrational energy. When violet appears in this part of the chart it is usually symbolic of the person who runs down the road with a sandwich in one hand and a can of drink in the other. They have no time to think of what they are eating or drinking and have no love of their digestive system. If they had they would change their eating habits.

MAGENTA If a person is eating something they are allergic to, this colour will appear in the metabolic section of the chart. It is indicating a need to eradicate this food from their diet in order for the body to return to its state of optimum health and vitality. If a person suspects that they have a food allergy, it is advisable to suggest that they attend a clinic which tests for these.

The Physical Aspect

RED-ORANGE When red-orange appears in this part of the spine it is indicating that there is a lack of physical energy, sometimes accompanied by a need for physical joy. This lack of energy might have resulted from a day of hard physical labour and if a good night's sleep is enjoyed it might not appear on a chart made the following day. Another reason for the appearance of this colour could be boredom or depression. When we are faced with the prospect of doing something that we really enjoy or spending time with a loved one, we experience a new lease of life and energy, but when confronted with loneliness or uninspiring work, boredom and lethargy arise. Another possible reason for this colour's appearance is that the person is not grounded — in other words, they are so heavenly minded they are no earthly good. If we are working towards wholeness, all aspects of ourselves have to be integrated.

GOLD This is the colour of wisdom and it appears in this part of the spine chart when a person lacks either the wisdom to take and follow the path in life which is most beneficial for them or the ability to select the right job or choose the appropriate place to live. Another trait that this colour reveals is an inability to learn from mistakes. Until a person has the wisdom to see the results of their mistakes they will keep repeating them. This can be likened to taking one step forward and two steps backwards. Wisdom is needed to move out of this rut.

YELLOW This colour's appearance in the physical aspect reveals a physically-orientated individual who gives little or no thought to the radiance which shines from their own inner light. Such people are usually impeccably dressed with not a hair out of place. This rather stern exterior could be a mask which covers a very fragile and unsure person. What we need to remember is that true beauty comes from within. If the eyes of a physically handicapped person radiate their inner light, for example, their physical deformities are barely noticed.

LIME GREEN Lime green in the physical part of the spine chart is either due to the presence of toxins in the body or a lack of physical balance. Toxicity in the body may be caused by an unwholesome diet or taking medication. One way of dealing with this is through a short fast taken when one is able to rest, followed by a change in diet. Anyone taking medication should not stop this without their doctor's consent but they can do a great deal to help themselves by being aware of the food they are eating and also by receiving complementary treatment regularly. A physical imbalance can be caused through the loss of an organ or limb or because parts of the body are not functioning to their full potential, leaving other parts with an increased workload. It could also be due to a diet that is either too acidic or too alkaline.

TURQUOISE Turquoise is the colour of immunity and when it appears in this part of the spine chart it could be indicating that the person is a hypochondriac. This is a well-known condition amongst student nurses and doctors. They attend lectures on various diseases and then start imagining that they have the symptoms described. The blue in this colour suggests that there is need for peace and relaxation in order that problems may be realistically addressed and mental and physical balance restored.

INDIGO This colour is a very powerful analgesic and its appearance on the physical aspect of the spine chart indicates that the person is suffering physical pain. With all pain, medical advice should be sought. Indigo is also a colour which creates space for silence and relaxation to be enjoyed. When this is related to the physical body it suggests the person needs these attributes to help them cope with a full and busy life. Our present-day lifestyle gives us relatively little time to enjoy the space and quietness so essential for our well-being.

VIOLET Violet in the physical is challenging us to ask how much love we have for our physical body, the temple of our soul. Many people, when asked if they love themselves, laugh and either answer 'no' or say that they are attempting to. Some have been conditioned that it is selfish and therefore wrong to love themselves, but as already mentioned, if they cannot do this, they cannot truly love anyone else. Another reason for people not loving their physical body is that they feel it is the wrong shape or size. This to me is not a good reason, because once we start to love our bodies, wonderful things start to happen.

MAGENTA Magenta is the colour which prompts a person to make changes so that they can evolve as human beings. When it appears in this part of the chart it is saying that the person needs to make changes in their physical life, perhaps by changing their job or giving up a sport or pastime that is no longer relevant. Whenever we give up something space is created for new ideas and pastimes to come in.

A Brief Interpretation of a Spine Chart

As an example of how to interpret a spine chart, let's look at the completed chart for 'Mrs A' in the Plate section. Starting at the top of the chart with the spiritual area, the colours of violet and indigo appear. Both of these colours are bridged, indicating that this person is working with the concept of unconditional love alongside searching for their own inner space. This inner space is usually found by practising meditation and following a spiritual discipline; a person with these two colours bridged is usually working with these.

Moving down into the mental area, the colours present are indigo and gold, which are bridged, and violet, which is unbridged. At this level the indigo is working to quieten the mind by stemming the constant stream of thoughts bombarding it and providing the space for the wisdom of the intuition (gold) to be acknowledged and listened to. This is only possible

Vertebral level/ Complementary colour	Body area	Conditions
1C / LG	Blood supply to the head, pituitary, scalp, facial bones, brain, inner and middle ear, sympathetic nervous system.	Headaches, nervousness, insomnia , head colds, hypertension, migraine, headaches, mental conditions, amnesia, epilepsy, tiredness, dizziness.
2C / Y	Eyes, optic nerve, auditory nerve, sinuses, mastoid bones, tongue, forehead.	Sinusitis, allergies, squint, deafness, crysipeias, eye troubles, earache, fainting spells, certain cases of blindness.
3C / GO	Cheeks, outer ear, face bones, teeth, trifacial nerve.	Neuralgia, neuritis, acne or pimples, eczema.
4C / RO	Nose, lips, mouth, eustachian tubes, adenoids.	Hayfever, catarrh, deafness, adenoid enlargement.
5C / M	Vocal cords, neck glands, pharynx.	Laryngitis, hoarseness, pharyngitis, quinsy, etc.
6C / V	Neck muscles, shoulders, tonsils.	Stiff neck, pain in upper arm, tonsillitis, whooping cough, croup.
7C / I	Thyroid gland, bursa in the shoulders, the elbows.	Bursitis, colds, thyroid conditions, goiters.
1D / T	Forearms, hands, wrists and fingers, the oesophagus and trachea.	Asthma, cough, difficult breathing, shortness of breath, pain in forearms and hands.
2D / LG	Heart, including its valves and covering, coronary arteries.	Functional heart conditions and certain chest pains.
3D / Y	Lungs, bronchial tubes, pleura, chest, breasts, nipples.	Bronchitis, pleurisy, congestion, pneumonia, influenza.
4D / GO	Gall bladder and common bile duct.	Gall bladder conditions, jaundice, shingles.
5D / RO	Liver, solar plexus, blood.	Liver conditions, fevers, low blood pressure, anaemia, poor circulation, arthritis.
6D / M	Stomach.	Stomach troubles including nervous stomach, indigestion, heartburn, dyspepsia, etc.
7D / V	Pancreas, islets of langerhans, duodenum.	Diabeties, ulcers, gastritis.
8D / I	Spleen, diaphragm.	Leukemia, hiccoughs, lowered resistance.
9D / T	Adrenals.	Allergies, hives.
10D / LG	Kidneys.	Kidney troubles, ateriosclerosis, chronic tiredness, nephritis, pyreitis.
11D / Y	Kidneys, ureters.	Skin conditions like acne or pimples, eczema, boils, etc. auto-intoxication.
12D / GO	Small intestines, fallopian tubes, lymph circulation.	Rheumatism, gas pains, certain types of sterility.
1L / RO	Large intestine (colon), inguinal rings.	Constipation, colitis, dysentery, diarrhoea, hernia.
2L / M	Appendix, abdomen, thighs, caecum.	Appendicitis, cramps, difficult breathing, acidosis, varicose veins.
3L / V	Sex organs, ovaries or testicles, uterus, bladder, knee.	Bladder troubles, menstrual troubles like painful or irregular periods, miscarriages, bed-wetting, impotence, menopause, knee pains.
4L / I	Prostate gland, muscles of the lower back, sciatic nerve.	Sciatica, lumbago, difficult, painful or too frequent urination.
5L / T	Legs, ankles, feet, heels, arches.	Poor circulation, weakness and cramps of the lower extremities, swollen ankles and arches, cold feet.
1S LG / 2S Y / 3S GO / 4S RO / 5S M / 1C V / 2C I / 3C T	— Hipbones, buttocks.	Sacro-iliac conditions, spinal curvature.
	— Rectum, anus.	Haemorrhoids, itching, pain at end of spine on sitting.

Every aspect of the body is controlled by nerves. Their normal function can be disturbed by vertebral misalignment, possibly effecting the disease conditions below.

Mental
air – human

throat chakra *

Emotional (Astral)
fire – animal

heart chakra *

Metabolic (Etheric)
water – plant

* solar plexus chakra

Physical
earth – mineral

* sacral chakra

* base chakra

Colour code
RO: red-orange
GO: gold
Y: yellow
LG: lime green
T: turquoise
I: indigo
V: violet
M: magenta

Medical colour – diagnosis chart and chart of the nervous system

97

when the mind is quiet and peaceful. If you refer back to the spiritual aspect of the chart you will see that this links with what is being worked with here in the mental. The challenge is the need to incorporate love and self-respect, shown by the unbridged violet.

The emotional aspect shows that a great deal is happening in this area of the person's life. The bridged magenta and yellow are showing an attempt to step back from day-to-day existence in order to learn what changes need to be made to create the freedom to walk forward. The emotional disturbances being experienced are producing a loss of emotional energy (red-orange) and a lack of emotional balance (green). These will have created an imbalance in both the astral layer of the aura and the solar plexus chakra.

The metabolic area is showing that this person is wisely looking at their diet (gold) and attempting to make it more nutritious, but is still eating something that is creating an allergic reaction (magenta). The lime green shows that the body is attempting to detoxify itself, but to complete this process the food that is causing the toxicity has to be found and eliminated.

In the physical areas the colours of indigo and red are both unbridged, showing that the person is lacking in physical energy and vitality, which could be due to their diet or their emotional problems, alongside the need to find more space for themselves.

The chakras on the chart which are not vibrating to the correct frequency are the sacral, the solar plexus and the throat. The overall colour needed to help the person find and work with the cause of their problems is red-orange.

Another way of working with this chart is to check it against the chart shown on page 97 to find which organs are connected to the nerves coming from the unbridged vertebrae. These organs can then be checked during a contact healing session for any stagnant energy (see Chapters 9 and 10). If stagnant energy is present, pearl is used, with visualisation, to help disperse it.

CHAPTER 7

DISEASE AND ITS METAPHYSICAL CAUSE

ONCE A DIAGNOSIS has been made, the first step towards healing is to examine the possible cause of the illness. These days we are conditioned into believing that illness is inflicted upon us by the outside world and if we are unfortunate enough to become ill then it is the medical profession who must take responsibility for our recovery. In saying this I am not decrying this profession, because I do believe that it has a necessary role to play in our present society, but I also believe that ultimately we have to be responsible for our own health or lack of it.

A basic goal in allopathic medicine is to discover how healing occurs. Up until now the belief has been that drugs or surgical procedures are responsible for this, but it is now gradually being accepted that consciousness may play a part in the effectiveness of all kinds of medical intervention.

Consciousness operates not only within a person but also operates between individuals and their states of consciousness can either help or hinder health. If we believe without doubt that we can overcome disease and are prepared to work with ourselves to find and eradicate the cause of the disease we will be cured. But if, through conditioning, we believe that we will die from a disease or we lack the will and courage to work with ourselves, then we most probably will die.

When running a course abroad, I met a remarkable lady. She had a mentally handicapped son and blamed herself for his disability. She had convinced herself that she should suffer for the plight of her son and then contracted breast cancer. When she discovered the breast lump she ignored it because she wanted to die. When she eventually decided to consult her

doctor her breast was solid with tumour. He showed no sympathy in informing her that she had acted irresponsibly and the tumour was now too
advanced for surgery.

At this point she realised that if she died there would be no one to look
after her son. On leaving the doctor's surgery she made a decision to inves-
tigate complementary therapies and sought treatment with the therapies she
felt drawn towards. With regular treatment and a conscious effort to recover,
she found that the lump started to diminish. When it had shrunk back to the
size it was when she first discovered it, she decided to have it removed surgically. After this she made a full recovery. Realising how much she had been
helped by complementary therapy and how effective these treatments are, she
trained as a therapist to enable herself to help others in the way she had been
helped.

If we have likewise chosen to work in the complementary medical field,
perhaps the questions we should be asking ourselves are: what is disease?
What is healing? How do we know if we have a high enough potential for
helping others to help themselves? If we have no plausible answers to these
questions, perhaps we should reconsider our path in life.

I personally believe that we are a minute speck in the vast universe surrounding us. I also believe that we ourselves are a mirror image of all that is
beyond ourselves. If we look at our planet we can see the devastation that is
occurring through pollution, chemicals and man's inhumanity towards his
fellow man as well as the animal and plant kingdom. All of this is manifesting in Earth changes and causing a variety of diseases to all life. To reverse
the horrors that are now taking place we have to root out the cause. We have
to stop polluting the Earth with chemicals and genetically modified food. We
have to respect all life, including the animal kingdom. Animals have their
own path of evolution and they are helped along this when they lose their
fear of man and learn to receive and give love. This certainly cannot happen
when we feel it is our right to experiment on these creatures for our so called
well-being or to kill them for their coats to beautify ourselves. We have a lot
of hard work to do if we are going to repair the harm that we have done
through the atrocities we have committed.

If we ourselves are a miniature universe, a microcosm of the macrocosm,
surely the same applies to us. Many people are now recognising motivation,
emotion and attitude as central to both health and disease. Among
disease-producing factors are stress, despair, deep unconscious fear and the

pollution of our own bodies with the food and drink we put into them. These factors, as already mentioned, create stagnant energy in the etheric layer of the aura. If this is not dealt with, it will eventually manifest as a physical disease. This leads me to believe that healing is related to the individual's willingness to find and work with the cause of the physically manifested disease. Failure to do this means they will not recover. But by working with the cause they themselves will take a step forward on life's evolutionary spiral and place themselves in a position where they are able to help others.

I see the physical body as a mirror reflecting where we stand and what we are doing on all levels of our being. It reflects our metaphysical condition through its systems and organs and the diseases which afflict them. Making practitioners aware of the metaphysical cause of some of these diseases gives them a greater understanding of their patients and the various ways in which they can be helped. It is also important to realise that disease can be a tremendous learning curve.

HOW OUR BODY SPEAKS TO US

The Head

Our head comprises the skull, which is formed from eight flat bones. These protect and house our brain, which is divided into a right and left hemisphere. The right hemisphere is connected to the left side of the body and the left hemisphere to the right side. The right hemisphere and left side of the body is associated with our feminine energy, our intuition and creativity, and the left hemisphere and right side of the body to our masculine energy, our intellect, logic and assertiveness. Our brain forms part of our nervous system and is the most complex and sophisticated electronic computer yet built. Like the rest of the body, the nervous system is vulnerable to various problems. It can be damaged by infections, degeneration, structural defects, tumours and vascular disorders caused by defects in its blood supply.

Our head contains our eyes, giving us our sense of sight, our ears for our sense of hearing, our mouth for our sense of taste and our nose for our sense of smell. So our head is our centre for thinking and sensing as well as being the control centre for the rest of the body. It is also related to our spiritual aspect.

Any diseases of the head can manifest through our desire to disconnect ourselves from the rest of our body or from our spirituality. The reasons for wanting to do this are many.

Amnesia (Loss of Memory)

This is usually caused by a blow to the head, which can damage the brain if forceful enough, but it can also occur for no apparent reason. Loss of memory can develop from deep emotional pain or trauma experienced during our childhood or in later years. The trauma here is so painful we cut ourselves off from it and the rest of the world. Doing this ensures that we will not have to endure a similar experience or remember the initial one.

Alzheimer's Disease

This condition affects quite a large percentage of the population. It is normally associated with old age but it can occur at any age. If it occurs before the age of 65 it is termed 'pre-senile' and after the age of 65 it is 'senile'. It is an incurable disorder of the brain in which there is a progressive loss of memory and other intellectual functions so that the mind gradually ceases to function normally and the affected person slowly becomes increasingly confused, incapable of sensible conversation and unaware of their surroundings. They often revert to childlike behaviour.

The metaphysical cause for this distressing condition could be deep mental trauma and/or an intense fear of the future. Reverting to childlike behaviour is one way of escaping from responsibility and avoiding having to face any fears or traumas that the future may hold. A child does not have to take responsibility for themselves, as this is done by their parents; likewise a person in the later stages of this disease is incapable of looking after themselves and this has to be done by either the family or an institution.

Headaches and Migraines

A headache can be a symptom of an underlying disorder, but it is more likely to be caused by stress, too little or too much sleep, overeating or drinking, or a noisy or stuffy environment. Physiologically, there are two causes for the pain in the head. The first is tension deriving from strain on facial, neck and scalp muscles and the second is the swelling of local blood vessels that results in strain within their walls.

A migraine is a severe headache which is preceded and accompanied by other symptoms. The biological cause is uncertain. Some neurologists believe a migraine is due to the way the arteries leading to the brain react to a triggering factor like chocolate or cheese, becoming first narrowed and then swollen. It is the narrowing of the arteries that reduces the blood supply to the brain. This could explain the blurred vision sometimes associated with this condition.

Metaphysically, headaches are caused through a mind that is overburdened with thoughts and feelings which cannot be expressed because of fear and through the pressures of work, relationships and family life. If you are someone who suffers from headaches, try to rationally look at your fears and the pressures that exist in your life. Unburden your mind by expressing what you are thinking and seek ways of relieving the pressures that are causing unease and tiredness.

The eyes

Our eyes are the windows of our soul and also the organs which allow us to assimilate our surroundings. If problems start to occur in our eyes the question we need to ask is: what don't we want to see?

Cataracts

A cataract is the gradual clouding up of the jelly-like substance that forms the lens of the eye. This blocks or distorts light entering the eye and so progressively distorts vision. In some cases this distortion is worse in bright sunlight. The question that arises here is: why do we not want to see clearly? What are we afraid or ashamed of that necessitates our hiding behind a dark cloud? The cloudy vision that a cataract gives prevents others from looking into the very soul of our being. A less drastic way of achieving the same result, one frequently adopted by young people, is to wear dark glasses whatever the weather.

Glaucoma

Glaucoma is one of the most common and severe eye disorders in people over 60. It is caused by a build up of aqueous humour due to a defective drainage system. This causes pressure to build up within the eyeball. The pressure causes the collapse and finally the death of tiny blood vessels at the back of the eye whose function is to nourish the nerve fibres of the optic disc.

Fluid is water, the element associated with our emotions. One way of expressing our feelings is through the tears of sorrow or tears of joy. A build up of aqueous fluid could indicate suppressed emotions that need to be released through crying. This is something that men living in the Western world find very difficult to do because they are conditioned into thinking that it is unmanly to cry.

The Ears

Our ears are the sense organs which allow us to hear and communicate with the sounds around us. Part of their construction are the semicircular canals which enable us to keep our balance. If we suffer ear problems we need to consider what it is that we don't wish to hear and where the imbalances are in our life.

Ménière's Disease

In this disease there is an increase in the amount of fluid in the labyrinth in the inner ear. This fluid-filled chamber constantly monitors the position and movement of the head and relays the information to the brain so that the body's balance can be maintained. The increased pressure caused by the excess fluid distorts or can rupture the nerve cells in the labyrinth wall, disturbing our sense of balance. This disease is challenging us to look at the imbalances in our life and to find ways of resolving them so that balance and harmony can be restored.

Ruptured Eardrum

The most common causes of this are a sharp object poked into the ear to relieve irritation, a blast from an explosion or a blow to the ear. A ruptured eardrum can lead to a partial loss of hearing. It is daring us to address those issues which we would prefer not to hear about, either because they involve doing something which we don't particularly like, or because we are afraid, or because the issues are too painful to look at. Whichever of these may be true, listening and acting on what we hear will enable us to walk forward with renewed strength and insight.

The Nose

This forms part of the respiratory tract. It is through the nose that we take in air to supply the body with the oxygen essential for energy production and to rid it of carbon dioxide, which is the waste product of energy production. From the nasal passages, pairs of air-filled cavities, the sinuses, branch into the bones of the skull. These reduce the weight of the head and give resonance to the voice.

Colds

The disease we call the common cold can be caused by any of nearly 200 different viruses. The symptoms of a runny, blocked nose are signs showing that we are cutting ourselves off from our higher intuitional self and that there are emotional issues which need to be addressed. A cold can give us the space needed to look at these issues and find the changes that need to be made to enable us to again flow freely with the energies of life.

Sinusitis

Sinusitis is inflammation of the mucous membrane lining the sinus cavities and usually develops as a complication of a virus infection such as a cold. It can also be triggered by dairy produce which irritates and encourages the membrane lining to secrete an excess of mucus. If we contract this condition we need to find what it is in our life that is irritating us. Irritation can create a build up of emotional anger which finds release through the sinuses if not dealt with.

The Neck

Our neck is the bridge between our physical and spiritual self. Within it is the larynx, which enables us to voice our opinions; the thyroid gland, which determines the body's metabolic rate through the production of the hormone thyroxine; and the parathyroids, which secrete parathyroid hormone, which, together with vitamin D, controls the level of calcium in the blood. Calcium is needed to strengthen our bones and our teeth, to clot blood and to enable our nerves and muscles to function.

Stiff Neck

If we suffer a stiff neck we are unable to move our head to view our surroundings, so we are only able to see what lies straight ahead. This could indicate that there is something in our life that we do not wish to look at or it could be symbolic of a very rigid and dogmatic mind. If we identify with either of these states, we need to gently remove our blinkers in order to see the whole and not just part of the reality surrounding us.

Laryngitis

This is usually caused by bacterial or viral infection and results in hoarseness or a complete loss of the voice. Our voice allows us to express our feelings and 'voice' our opinions and beliefs. If we lose our voice, we are unable to do this and we need to ask ourselves the reason why. It may be through fear of being ridiculed for what we believe or fear of being laughed at, or we may consider ourselves unworthy to be a part of the company we find ourselves in. What is important to remember is that our feelings are a very important part of us and there are times when they need to be voiced.

Hyperthyroidism (Overactive Thyroid)

This is a condition in which excessive amounts of thyroxine are produced. This causes a general speeding up of all chemical reactions in the body, which affects mental as well as physical processes. This process mirrors a stressful and agitated individual who is trying to reach their aims in life too quickly, often to the detriment of the people surrounding them. They want everything to be completed before it has started. They are trying to run faster than their legs will carry them. The physical body itself shows this by accelerating the ageing process and the deterioration of the body.

Hypothyroidism (Underactive Thyroid)

This is caused when the thyroid gland produces too little thyroxine, resulting in the slowing down of the body's metabolism. The result is tiredness, general aches and pains and a slowing down of the heart rate. This disease can show a lethargic personality that has very little desire to enter into anything, an attitude which says, 'I can't be bothered, life really isn't worth living.' If this is true then the individual needs to be jolted out of it by being constantly reminded that they have come to Earth for a purpose, a purpose that they need to find and fulfil.

The Shoulders and Arms

The shoulder is connected to the upper arm by a ball and socket joint. The ball of the upper arm bone fits into a cup-shaped socket in the shoulder blades. Our shoulders are where we carry the burdens and responsibilities of life and our arms are used to show our feelings for our fellow human beings and to express how we are feeling about things in general.

A Frozen Shoulder

A frozen shoulder is one in which the normal range of movement is impossible because of stiffness and pain. This condition usually starts with a minor injury which affects use of the joint. In severe cases the pain can travel down the corresponding arm. If we suffer this, we need to look at the burdens and responsibilities we are carrying. Have we become frozen under their weight and so rigid that we are no longer able to express how we feel about ourselves and others? If so, it is time to look at these burdens and lay down those which are no longer relevant so that we can again open our arms to free expression. One of the failings of some practitioners is taking on their patients' burdens. This is no help to the practitioner or to the patient. The patient fails to learn and the practitioner eventually becomes sick.

The Chest

Encased within the protective ribcage are the lungs, which are connected with the breath of life, and the heart, which is the centre of love and emotional harmony. In a female the mammary glands are also found here. These symbolise the caring and nurturing feminine energy.

Breast Cancer

This is the most serious disorder of the breast but one that can be successfully treated by conventional medicine if diagnosed in its early stages. The breasts are where we nurture the newborn infant and as women use our nurturing energy for the rest of our family. If we nurture others, we ourselves need to be nurtured, but for a lot of women this never happens and the body shows this through breast-related diseases. Breast diseases can also be an outward manifestation of inner conflicts related to a denial of the feminine energy by men and the important role this energy plays in our present society.

Coronary Heart Disease

This condition occurs when the two coronary arteries, which nourish the heart by means of a network of branches over its surface, become narrowed with fatty deposits. This causes angina, which can lead to a heart attack. The heart is the centre where we give and receive love, and our inability to do either of these manifests physically as heart disease. As well as giving and receiving love we have to learn to love ourselves. The laying down of fatty deposits in the two coronary arteries is a form of protection against 'heartache' and a 'broken heart', but unfortunately this process becomes detrimental to the heart by starving it of the right amount of oxygen and food needed for its physical function. The first step towards healing heart disease is to love every aspect of ourselves. This leads to the second step which is to radiate unconditional love to all of creation.

Asthma

Asthma is a condition marked by frequent and sustained attacks of breath-lessness. The cause is a partial obstruction of the bronchi and bronchioles, which is due to contraction of their wall muscles. Asthmatics are expressing a difficulty in being at ease in the world. They may feel they are not living up to expectations or fear rejection because they believe they are not good enough. To overcome this we first have to learn to accept ourselves. If we can do this we will automatically be accepted by other people.

Bronchitis

Bronchitis is inflammation of the mucous lining of the main air passages of the lungs and usually caused by the same viruses that cause colds. When we develop a cough or inflamed bronchial tissues we are often expressing our inner frustration or irritation with how we are feeling about ourselves. It may indicate that we need to get something off our chest, that something we are trying to say has become blocked. There may be issues from deep within us that are starting to surface, but we have not yet developed the courage or means to confront them. The condition may also relate to irritation connected with either events or experiences in our personal life that is making it hard for us to breathe in deeply.

The Upper Abdomen

This part of the body houses our main digestive organs, namely our stomach, liver, gall bladder, spleen and pancreas. It is related to the element of fire due to the heat and energy produced during the process of digestion.

The Stomach

The stomach acts as a food reservoir and processor, transforming the bulk of a chewed and swallowed meal into a slow trickle of pulp. This processed food then trickles out of the stomach through the pyloric sphincter into the duodenum.

Obesity

Obesity is carrying a surplus of fat through overindulgence in food. Food represents the mother, love, affection, security, survival and reward. We use it to replace affection and love, especially at times of loss, separation or death to try and fill the emptiness within.

Gastric Erosion

A gastric erosion is a raw area in the mucous membrane that lines the stomach. It can be caused by certain drugs that irritate the membrane or by prolonged emotional stress. Instead of the stomach digesting the food put into it for our benefit, it is itself being eroded. This usually stems from emotional issues that we are 'unable to stomach'. Here we are being seriously challenged to look at our life to find a way of resolving these issues.

The Liver

The liver is the largest single organ in the body and plays a crucial and complex role in regulating the composition of various chemicals and cells in the blood. It is very much associated with love and lovability. It governs love/hate relationships and is the organ where anger is stored. Broken homes profoundly affect the liver at a psychic level.

Cirrhosis of the Liver

Cirrhosis is the slow deterioration of the liver due to gradual internal scarring. These changes make the liver progressively less able to carry out its numerous and vital functions. The scars the liver bears can be caused by an excess of alcohol taken to numb anger we carry towards ourselves as well as the anger engendered by the actions of other people. If our liver is to remain healthy, we have to express our anger and remedy its cause.

Acute Hepatitis

Acute hepatitis is a sudden inflammation of the liver caused by one of several viruses. Three of these have been identified and have been termed A, B and C. Hepatitis A is spread from person to person when food or water is contaminated or by poor personal hygiene. Both hepatitis B and hepatitis C are spread from person to person by two main routes: contact with infected blood and sexual activities. Victims of hepatitis C are particularly likely to develop chronic liver disease.

Our liver is able to handle very heavy stress but if it becomes inflamed it is showing that our stress levels are so high that it can no longer cope, making it susceptible to infection. Our liver also carries or senses biorhythms and the rhythm of the Earth, enabling the human organism to be put in touch with its own natural biorhythms. When the liver becomes inflamed, the sense of these biorhythms is lost to the human body.

The Gall Bladder

The gall bladder is a collecting bag for fluid containing bilirubin and various other substances. It lies on the surface of the liver. After a meal, it empties its contents, called bile, along the bile duct into the duodenum.

This small organ has a descriptive language that tells us clearly what is going on. Gall is usually associated with guts or courage, but also irritation and insensitivity. Bile is associated with bitterness. Therefore gall bladder problems can be linked to emotional and mental patterns of irritation and bitterness towards other people or with situations in our life which upset us.

Gallstones

Gallstones are stones which form in the gall bladder. A gallstone starts as a tiny solid particle which grows as more material solidifies around it. So our thought patterns may congeal and harden, becoming gallstones that may be very difficult to release. The power of negative thought is not to be underestimated.

The Pancreas

The pancreas is a long thin gland that lies crosswise just behind the stomach. It has two major functions. The first is to produce enzymes which flow through the pancreatic duct into the duodenum, where they help to digest food. The second is to produce the hormones insulin and glycogen, which play an important part in regulating the glucose level in the blood.

Diabetes Mellitus

This is a common disorder caused by a deficiency or total lack of insulin production by the pancreas. This results in a low absorption of glucose – both by the cells that need it for energy and by the liver that stores it – and consequently in a high level of glucose in the blood. There are two main forms of diabetes. They are type one, known as juvenile onset or insulin dependent diabetes, and type 2, known as maturity onset or insulin independent diabetes.

Suffering from diabetes is inviting us to look at our inability to be kind or sweet to others. In the same way that glycogen has to be balanced in our physical body so the kindness and sweetness that we confer on ourselves and others has likewise to be balanced. To be 'sugary sweet' is to exude sweetness which is neither balanced, beneficial or appreciated by other people. The opposite end of the spectrum is where sweetness and kindness have been replaced by sourness and bad humour!

The Spleen

The spleen is essentially a very large lymph gland lying on the upper left side of the abdomen. In addition to producing lymphocytes, it also removes old and malformed red cells from the bloodstream and breaks them down.

The Chinese believe that the energising of our spleen by *prana* entering its two minor chakras gives us our sense of humour and a zest for living but it is made weak through self-denial and by avoiding meeting our responsibilities. Sufferers frequently wear masks to cover their true feelings and to give themselves some form of immunity to outside influences.

Enlarged Spleen

The spleen nearly always becomes enlarged as a symptom of another disorder. An enlarged spleen sometimes becomes overactive in removing various types of cells from the blood and is also prone to rupture. It carries the feelings hidden behind the masks we wear and the responsibilities we are trying to avoid or become immune to. Accepting the challenges that responsibilities bring leads us to further strength and wisdom.

The Lower Abdomen

The lower abdomen houses the small intestine, colon, bladder, kidneys, adrenal glands, uterus, ovaries and testes.

Small Intestine

The small intestine is approximately 5m long and runs between the duodenum and the colon. Its main function is the absorption of nutrients into the bloodstream.

The small intestine is greatly affected by our instinctive flight or fight reactions and adrenal activity. It registers fear and anything that would appear to be threatening. It is also involved in the registration of sound waves.

Crohn's Disease

Crohn's disease is a chronic inflammation of part of the digestive tract. The part most commonly affected is the ileum, although patches of inflammation can occur anywhere. Inflammation along any part of the intestinal tract is an indication that we are absorbing instead of facing and resolving the things we fear or are threatened by. When we become afraid, the adrenal glands secrete greater quantities of adrenaline into the bloodstream which, when not used to extricate ourselves from imminent danger, remain in the physical body, causing hyperactivity.

The Colon

The colon or large intestine is approximately 1.5m in length. The small intestine opens into the large intestine through a pouch-like chamber called the caecum. The rest of the colon then runs up the right side of the body, across under the ribcage and down the left side of the body, forming a cage for the small intestine.

The colon is associated with guilt and conditions of conscience. People who tell themselves they are bad also damage their colon. The colon deals with our unwanted emotions and our inability to express these as well as emotions of attachment. The fact that there is so much bowel dysfunction nowadays points very strongly to the fact that people cannot let go of their emotional attachments, good or bad, and stand free.

Constipation

This is a condition in which the bowels are opened infrequently or incompletely, as a result of which the stools are dry and hard. If we suffer constipation we have to look at our emotional attachments and question why we are frightened to let go of them. The reason could be insecurity or conditioning. However painful, holding on will deny us the freedom to become our own master.

Diarrhoea

Diarrhoea is increased frequency, fluidity or volume of bowel movements as compared to a person's customary pattern of bowel movement. On a physical level, diarrhoea can be caused through food poisoning and is the body's way of eliminating the organisms involved as quickly as possible. Metaphysically, this condition is the body's way of quickly ridding itself of negative emotions before they create disharmony within the physical body.

The Kidneys

The kidneys are a pair of glands situated close to the spine in the upper part of the abdomen. Their chief function is to separate fluid and certain solids from the blood. When the kidneys fail, the solid waste substances accumulate in the blood. The resulting 'poisoning' produces the clinical condition known as uraemia. Our kidneys register agitation, hatred, anxiety and emotional discord and will work to rid the system of these feelings.

Kidney stones

A kidney stone normally begins as a tiny speck of solid matter deposited in the middle of the kidney where urine collects before flowing into the ureter.

As further bits of material cling to the first speck, it gradually builds into a solid mass. A kidney stone can be an accumulation of anxiety or hatred that has not been resolved. The longer the condition continues, the larger the stone becomes.

The Bladder

The bladder is a sac formed of muscular and fibrous tissue and lined by a mucous membrane. Its function is to collect the urine passed down the ureter tubes from the kidneys. The bladder is very much connected with child-like emotions and is very sensitive to seasonal changes. The bladder meridian, which passes through the bladder, is involved in the flow of the kundalini energy up the spine. If this meridian is blocked, it hampers the flow of the kundalini energy and reduces our physical vitality.

Cystitis

Cystitis is inflammation of the bladder and is normally caused by infection. If we are unable to release our child-like emotions through crying, the body attempts to release them through urine. Failure to do this results in the bladder becoming inflamed. It is known that some women can suffer from this condition through seasonal changes, showing their unwillingness to change certain aspects of their life.

The Ovaries

The ovaries form part of a women's reproductive system and are connected with her menstrual cycle, which is governed by the cycles of the moon. These glands produce the ova capable, if fertilised, of developing into a new human being. The ovaries are an expression of a woman's feminine power and creativity, and can suffer from disease when this power is undermined and her creativity on all its various levels is suppressed.

Ovarian Cyst

An ovarian cyst is a sac full of fluid which grows on or near an ovary. It occurs for no physical reason and can grow to a considerable size and interfere with fertility. It may also affect the menstrual cycle and prevent conception, both of which can metaphysically be caused through a suppression of female energy. The cyst is an accumulation of the conflicts and doubts which some women feel towards their feminine energy. Such feelings could stem from childhood sexual abuse which understandably has been too painful and traumatic to deal with.

The Uterus

The uterus is a pear-shaped organ whose walls are composed of powerful muscles. At its lower front end is a narrow thick-walled neck, the cervix, which leads into the top of the vagina. The uterus is the feminine expression of power and creativity and is a part of the unique reproductory system which distinguishes a woman from a man. The uterus also serves as a hollow-sounding chamber which vibrates to the primordial sounds of the universe.

Fibroids

Fibroids are benign tumours of the uterus which develop either within the muscular wall of the uterus or on the outside or inside wall, attached by a stalk of tissue. They can interfere with conception and gestation. If a woman develops this complaint she is doubting her feminine role and mistrusting her ability to carry and nurture a new life. This may be through the fear and doubt that a woman sometimes has about her own energy and the important role that this plays in the evolution of mankind.

The Testes

The testes, the male sex organs, hang suspended outside the body in a pouch of skin called the scrotum. Each gland is attached to the body by a single spermatic cord which is composed of the vas deferens and a number of nerves and blood vessels. The sperm produced by each testicle remain in a coiled tube, the epididymis, to mature. From here they pass into the vas deferens and seminal vesicles for storage. Problems relating to the male reproductive organs can stem from doubt and fear of not being able to sire children. The inability to do this often undermines a man's masculinity and his conditioned role in life.

Testicular Cancer

Cancer in this part of the body is the result of feelings of hopelessness and inadequacy centred around the male role. These feelings, if not faced and resolved, may become so deeply embedded that they start to eat away the physical body in the form of cancer. Whether we have incarnated in a male or female body, it is important to remember that both these energies should complement each other with the recognition that each has a vital role to play.

The Legs

Our legs comprise the thigh bone, knee joint, the tibia and fibula, and the ankle joint which attaches our feet to our legs. Our legs are the part of our anatomy which allow us to move from one place to another and our knees allow greater flexibility in several planes of movement. If we have problems with our legs we have to look at why we are resisting walking forward in life, preferring to stay stuck. Knee problems challenge us to examine whether or not we are working with our spiritual or ego self.

Rheumatoid Arthritis of the Knee

Rheumatoid arthritis is a long-term disease of the joints. The synovial membrane of the joint gradually becomes inflamed and swollen and this leads to inflammation of other parts of the joint. The swelling and inflammation prevents us from bending the joint to kneel down. What this is challenging us to see is whether we are working from our ego for self-glorification or with the humility that comes from our higher self. If we are working from the ego it will restrict and confine the work we do and prevent us from flowing with the energies of life. To remedy this we should remind ourselves that our gifts are not really ours but given to us by the universal light to use for the good of others. If we are able to accept this then we will carry out our tasks in life with humility and grace.

Leg Cramp

Cramp is a spasm in a muscle and can be caused by prolonged periods of sitting, standing or lying in an uncomfortable position. If we suffer leg cramp it can be connected to our inability to walk forward in life through fear or stubbornness. It is indicating that we have been standing in the same space for too long. Our growth and understanding of life depend upon our ability to move forward into new pastures.

OTHER CAUSES OF DISEASE

When we work as complementary practitioners, knowing the metaphysical interpretation of physical diseases allows us to look at our patients on another level of understanding, but not all diseases necessarily stem from a metaphysical cause. If we trip over and break our leg perhaps the lesson we have to learn is to be more careful. Disease can also be karmic. This means that the person has chosen to either incarnate with a physical disease or disability or to contract one later on in life. If the cause is karmic and the soul has chosen to die through their disease, then it will not be cured. The role of the practitioner in these cases is to help the person to die with dignity, free from fear. Remember that death is the ultimate cleanser and healer. Each one of us incarnates with the purpose of paying off a set amount of karma and the way chosen to do this is very individual.

CHAPTER 8

※

PROTECTION AND CLEANSING

BEFORE STARTING to work with patients, it is useful for therapists to give some thought to their own protection. The dictionary's definition of 'protection' is 'to shield the physical body from danger, injury, loss or harm'. Hopefully, as therapists, we will have no need to do this, in which case what are we protecting and why? The answer is we are protecting our physical, psychic and spiritual energies from being drained by those we come into contact with.

The greater our sensitivity, the greater our need to protect these energies. I have frequently heard sensitive people complain that they feel drained of all energy after shopping in a crowded city or attending a football match or concert. The truth is they *have* been drained of energy. Quite unknowingly and unwittingly, much of the crowd has acted like blotting paper, soaking up the energy of a percentage of the more sensitive people. They do this by projecting thread-like tentacles into people's auras and then siphoning off their energy. I am sure there have been times when you have been in the company of a patient or friend who has unburdened their problems to you. As they are about to leave they thank you for listening and remark how much better they are feeling, but leave you feeling completely drained of energy. Unfortunately they have filled their energy gap with your energy. If this were to happen on a regular basis, you would soon become ill.

All living entities are surrounded by an electromagnetic field, or aura, and when our energy field comes into contact with another field a vibration is sent through it. This vibration is eventually picked up by our nervous system and interpreted as either negative or positive. The same reaction occurs with the energies present in buildings, the countryside and places of exceptional beauty. The art of protection is to become aware of these energies in order to absorb those which are beneficial and shut out those which are not. I have heard it argued that we should learn to 'bind' the negative energies of our fellow human beings to stop them being projected at us. I personally feel that this is wrong and see it as a subtle form of manipulation. Our task is learning to become the master of our own energies, not the energies of our fellow human beings.

METHODS OF PROTECTION

The method or methods used for protection are very much an individual choice. What works for one person may not be so effective for another. Therefore it is a good idea to read about the various methods given in this chapter and in other books on the subject and select the one you feel attracted towards and feel will work for you. At a later date you may wish to work with other techniques or use a different protection for individual situations.

However you choose to work, it is important to remember to protect yourself at the start of each day. When I had qualified as a colour practitioner through the Maitreya School and was working alongside Lily Cornford, she continually asked me if I had protected myself. One day I told her that I believed that if we were working with universal energies for the good of others we would automatically be protected. She stopped what she was doing, turned to face me and said, 'My dear child, God helps those that help themselves'. I didn't realise the full implication of what she had said at the time but I certainly do now. If we were automatically protected by the higher power of the universal light, our power of free will would be taken away and we would never learn to become our own master.

The Equi-Limbed Cross of Light within a Circle of Light

This very potent sign has been used from earliest times and is still in use today. The equi-limbed cross refers to the four quarters of the globe and the four elements of earth, water, air and fire; it signifies God's dominion over these and occultly formulates His kingdom within the work of the operator (see opposite).

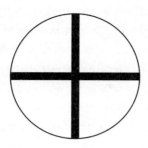

The equi-limbed cross

A very sensitive part of the body where the drainage of energy takes place is the solar plexus. To prevent this happening, the cross of light contained within a circle of light is traced with the fingers over this part of the body before going into a crowd and before treating a patient.

This will help you to avoid picking up the patient's disharmonies and taking them into your own body as well as prohibiting any drainage of your energies. If you forget to do this before the patient enters the therapy room, mentally visualise it when they are present. To make the sign of the cross and the circle, the first and second fingers of the right hand are extended; the third and fourth fingers are bent towards the palm of the hand and the thumb is laid across their nails.

Another reason for sealing our solar plexus is to seal the emotional or astral plane of our being. This prevents our own emotions obstructing the flow of healing energy and raises our vibrational energy to the mental and spiritual plane, where our focus should be, especially if we are working with colour contact healing.

To empower this sign, the following mantra can be said while tracing it on your solar plexus:

'Before me is Raphael,
Behind me is Uriel,
On my right stands Michael,
On my left stands Gabriel,
For around me flames the pentagram and in the centre stands the
column with the six-pointed star.'

Gabriel, Raphael, Michael and Uriel are four of the archangels responsible for bringing messages from the universal light to mankind. They give us light, strength, love and inspiration for use in everyday life. Gabriel is the messenger for the word of God and helps us to find our own inner truth, talents and gifts. Raphael is the angel of healing, responsible for healing the Earth and its inhabitants. Michael is the warrior whose light triumphs over the darkness of negativity and helps us find our own inner light. Uriel is the regent of the sun, helping us to acknowledge the light within all people and to become strong channels for the healing energy of the universe to flow through.

The pentagram symbolises the figure of a man with outstretched arms and legs. Like the circle, it has the power to bind negative energies. The six-pointed star depicts the creation. It is the combination of the masculine and feminine energies and the triangles of fire and water.

Visualisation Using a Sheet of Plate Glass

When counselling people whose energies overwhelm you, visualise them separated from you by a sheet of plate glass. You can see and hear through this, but others' magnetism cannot reach you. Visualise this sheet of glass until it appears to you to be absolutely tangible.

This visualisation can be used when working with the colour therapy instrument (see pages 171–3). When using this machine it is important to stay in the room with the patient but not to absorb the colour and complementary colour they are being treated with. This could have an adverse effect upon you, especially if you were treating several patients in a day, each with a different colour. To protect yourself from the vibrational energies of these colours, visualise a sheet of plate glass between you and the colour therapy instrument. This allows you to interact with the patient but stops the colours penetrating you.

Protection When Counselling

A method of protecting yourself when counselling someone who you feel saps your vitality is to sit on a chair with both feet in contact with each other on the floor. Interlace your fingers and place your folded hands across your solar plexus, keeping your elbows pressed against your sides. This posture makes your body a closed circuit, preventing the loss of any of your own energy.

Cloaking Protections

The first of these is visualising yourself putting on a cloak which is blue on the inside but steel grey on the outside. This cloak reaches down to the ground, has a hood to cover your head and a zip fastener up the front. Each time you safely wrap yourself in your cloak its blue lining gives you a wonderful sense of peace and tranquillity but its grey exterior stops the penetration of all negative energies.

A second way of cloaking yourself is with a pair of golden wings. Imagine that you have a large pair of golden wings radiating out from your back. When you feel the presence of negative energy or you feel the need for protection in any given situation, gently fold your wings across your body.

Another method you might try is to create for yourself a protective bubble. With each inhalation, breathe in golden light until this fills your body from head to toe. Then, with each exhalation, imagine this golden light being squeezed out of the pores of your body into your aura until you become encapsulated in a beautiful bubble of golden light. In a similar way to the sheet of plate glass, you are able to see and project out from your protective bubble, but nothing or no one can enter it unless you choose to invite them in.

One of my students had a very interesting experience with this visualisation. Most weekends her grandson visits her and enjoys sitting on her lap to be read a story. Prior to his coming she had protected herself with this method, as was her custom each day. When her grandson arrived he climbed on to her lap and then started to scream and fought with her to stand down. She was very distressed and had no explanation as to why this had happened. It was not until she attended her next weekend course and related this story that she understood the reason why. Children are very sensitive to people's energies and through protecting herself with a bubble of golden light, she had 'shut out' her grandson and he did not like this feeling. If she had been aware of this, she could have visualised a door opening in her protective bubble to allow her grandson in.

The Use of Salt and Water

Salt and water are both powerful mediums for absorbing negative energy and for purification. Salt is a crystalline structure able to absorb any negative energies surrounding it. It is the emblem of the element of earth and related to the physical and astral bodies.

In Graeco-Roman times salt played an important role in sacrifices and was also apotropaic, being placed on the lips of Roman infants when they were eight days old to ward off evil spirits. Today it is still a Japanese custom to scatter salt in a house that has entertained anyone with negative energies.

Water is the counterpart of light and has the power to dissolve, purify and infuse new life. In baptism, it is used to wash away the old life and sanctify the new. In the same way that light pierces the darkness of negativity, fear and hatred and guides us towards the positive, water, which is liquid light, will wash any negativity away.

CLEANSING OURSELVES OF NEGATIVITY

Sometimes, if we have had a particularly busy day treating people who are surrounded by a lot of negativity, we may feel that we have attracted some of this energy to ourselves. One way to remedy this is to take a salt bath.

Whenever we take a bath or a shower the intention is important. If we are bathing purely to cleanse the physical body, then only this part of us will be cleansed but if it is our intention to cleanse our aura as well, then this will happen. If we are taking a bath to cleanse ourselves of any negativity we may have contracted during the course of the day, it is good to make it into a ritual, bearing our intent in mind.

Method

When you have run the bath, have ready in a small container two table-spoons of salt to drop into the water. The ideal salt to use is block salt from mines. Failing this, sea salt can be used, but due to pollution, these salts are no longer pure. To bless the salt and water the following procedure can be adopted:

STEP 1: SAY THE GAYATRI:

O thou who givest sustenance to the universe,
From whom all things proceed,
To whom all things return,

Unveil to us the face of the true spiritual sun,
Hidden by a disc of golden light,
That we may know the truth
And do our whole duty
As we journey to Thy sacred feet.

STEP 2

Pouring the salt into the bath, make the sign of the equi-limbed cross over the salt and the water. Say a blessing three times over them invoking the specific qualities you require (e.g. qualities for cleansing, purification or for protection). In saying the blessing three times, the first time we are requesting the blessing we have asked for, the second time the energies created from the blessing start to infiltrate the water and the third time the blessing becomes sealed in the water. When doing this, your hand should be held flat over the bathwater with the fingers together and the thumb positioned at right angles to the forefinger.

All that remains for you to do now is to get into the bath and enjoy it.

Salt water which has been blessed can be placed in a small bowl in your therapy room to dip your fingers in when treating a patient with a serious illness or with an aura that is congested with stagnant energy. Dipping fingers into the salted water will cleanse them of any accumulated energy picked up from the patient.

Prior to treating a patient with severe negativity, place in your therapy room a bowl of blessed salted water next to a lighted candle. This will give protection to yourself and the patient. When treating patients with serious diseases like cancer and AIDS, it is recommended that you wash your hands and arms, up to the elbow, in salt water.

THE POWER OF PRAYER

The power of prayer is something which should never be overlooked. Whatever situation we find ourselves in we should always be able to visualise a cross of light and call upon the name of the Christ energy if we follow the Christian tradition, or a sacred symbol and the name of a deity concerned with whatever religion or esoteric path that we follow. The force of universal light and love is a balancing, healing, redeeming and purifying energy and should be invoked where any human element, incarnate or discarnate, is concerned.

My own experience of the power of prayer stems back many years. I was practising meditation early one morning when I became aware of a dark presence in the room with me. I immediately visualised a cross of light between it and me and it quickly dissolved.

BEING GROUNDED

To work with people, especially in a healing context, we have to be grounded, to have both our feet placed firmly on the Earth, and to be fully integrated with our physical body. If we are not, we are susceptible to negative energies and do not make a very good channel because this involves working with both the Earth energies and spiritual energies. The following exercise is one you might try practising if you feel the need to be grounded.

Grounding exercise

Either stand bare-foot on the earth or visualise yourself doing this. Imagine yourself to be like a tree with thick roots burrowing deep into the earth and with branches lifting into the light of the sun.

On your next inhalation, bring a shaft of white light through your crown chakra and imagine it flowing through your body via the other major chakras, down your legs and into your feet. As you exhale, see this energy passing from your feet into your imaginary roots which take it deep into the earth. On your next inhalation, draw the earth energy through your roots, into your feet and back up your body to your head where, on the next exhalation, it passes back into the universe through your crown chakra.

If you need to be grounded but do not have the time to work with the above technique, put some rock salt into your pocket. This will give you an 'earth' connection.

FINDING OUR OWN SPACE

When people are constantly dealing with and surrounded by other human beings, it is vital that they find space to feel into themselves and their own energy field. Only when we sit quietly in our own space can we check our own energy levels and our aura for any negativity we may have attracted to us and make sure that we are properly grounded. This is a bit like checking the store cupboard to see if anything needs replenishing. The following visualisation exercise is to help you to create your own inner space where you can rest and reflect upon yourself.

Creating our inner room

Sitting quietly and comfortably in a place where you will not be disturbed, bring your concentration to your breath. Make your inhalation the same length as your exhalation. This will help you to relax and quieten your mind from the constant bombardment of thoughts.

When you feel ready, visualise yourself standing in a corridor at the end of which is a door. Start to walk towards the door and when you reach it push it open and walk through into a room. This room can take on any form or shape you would like it to be.

Look round your room and visualise where you would like any windows to be placed and if you would like patio doors, visualise them and the outdoor scene you would like to see through them. Next, decorate the ceiling and put in place a ceiling light if you would like one. Move on to the walls, which you can either paper or paint in your favourite colours. When you have completed this, decide what you would like to cover the floor with and what colour this will be. Now look at any windows in your room and drape them with curtains or blinds. Lastly, put into your room anything that pleases you. These could be, for example, items of furniture, scatter cushions, candles, incense or a small water fountain.

Now stand back and look at your creation. If there is anything that you would like to change or add, then do it.

What you have just created is your own imaginary room where you can retreat to at will, a place where you can be completely alone or if you wish to be with a particular person, imagine them there with you. Whenever you feel the need for space, sit quietly and imagine yourself back in your own special room.

CLEANSING

Cleansing is the act of clearing a house, room or space of negative energies. This is sometimes necessary when we move house or when we have treated a particularly negative or sick patient. Keeping our therapy room physically clean is extremely important. Not all sensitive patients protect themselves and it is these patients who are most likely to pick up negative energies left by earlier patients.

Simple methods for cleaning a house of a bad psychic atmosphere is to strew garlic about the place, leave it overnight then collect it and burn it the next day.

Roses and mint in the house act as a general antiseptic against psychic influences, their perfumes and that of freesias are good for maintaining positive psychic energy and helping to dispel negative psychic energy.

If a room in the house has a particularly bad energy, place a large amethyst at its centre and leave it there with the door closed for a week, or even a month if the energy is very bad. During this time, the room should be left undisturbed. When you eventually return you may find that the crystal has lost its colour and will appear to be almost white. If you now bury it in the earth for approximately three months, it will be cleansed and its colour restored. (If you do bury it, it is a good idea to place a marker at the site so that you can easily locate it.)

Another method for cleansing a house or room is to prepare a bowl of salt water and bless it as described on page 124. Then, dipping your hands into the solution, splash some in each corner of the room or rooms and make the sign of the equi-limbed cross of light. Now make the sign of this cross with the salt water on the inside and outside of every door. Finally, make this sign with the salt water in the centre of the room or, if you are cleaning a house, in the centre of all the rooms, including the attic and the cellar. Having completed this cleansing, you might like to burn good-quality joss sticks around the house.

For those of you who prefer to work with visualisation, go into the room that needs cleansing and visualise a piece of violet material covering the floor area. Now imagine this piece of material starting to float upwards towards the ceiling, collecting within it all negative energies. When it nears the ceiling, visualise four angels, one placed at each corner, gathering the cloth together, taking it out through a window and burning it on a fire.

Protecting by cutting the ties that bind

When two people have been in a close relationship, ties or cords are formed uniting them. These are the same ties which bond a mother and child. They resemble very thin, flexible tubes through which energy flows. They stem from either the heart, the solar plexus or from both, depending on the nature of the relationship. A mother and child, for example, would form ties from the heart. It is along these ties that two people interact with each other at a psychic level and the longer the relationship has existed, the greater their strength.

The ties can be of a positive or negative nature. Positive ties exist between people who care for and respect each other, but these can turn negative when a relationship ends but one of the partners tries to hold on to the other. Another example would be a mother who tries to possess her adult son, sometimes to the detriment of his own family. Under normal circumstances, once a relationship has ended these ties slowly disintegrate unless two people choose to keep them intact through friendship.

If, after a relationship has ended, one partner is conscious that they are being influenced by the other and finds that the protection techniques described in this chapter are not helping, then the ties that bind can be consciously severed through visualisation. This enables both parties to walk free and continue with their own lives. The visualisation given below is one technique that you may find helpful.

Cutting Ties

Imagine that you are sitting in front of a deep indigo crystal. As you concentrate upon the crystal, it starts to grow. When it has reached the size of a small room, stand up and walk round it to look for a door. When you have found one, push it open and walk through into a crystal room bathed in indigo light.

Looking around the room you notice two chairs facing each other. Walk over to the chair that is on your left-hand side and sit there quietly for a few moments. Allow the indigo rays of light to penetrate your being to release any tension or fear that you might have.

When you feel relaxed and calm, visualise the person with whom you wish to cut the ties entering the crystal room through a door opposite to the one where you entered. See them walking across the room and sitting down on the chair that is facing yours. Look to see where the ties that bind you stem from and how thick these are.

On the floor to the right of your chair is a large bag containing a number of tools, including a pair of scissors and a saw as well as a large jar of healing balm. Taking the appropriate instrument, cut the ties that bind you. When you have done this, place the instrument back in the bag. Now take hold of the ends of your ties and pull out their roots from inside you. When you have done this, invite the person sitting opposite to do the same. If they choose not to do this, then it is ok. They can no longer affect you.

Next take the jar of healing balm and rub it into the wound left by your roots before handing it to the other person, if they have chosen to remove their roots.

Finally visualise the person that you have just cut ties with surrounded in a protective orb of golden light. Watch as they stand up and walk back out of their door of entry.

When they have gone, pick up the roots that you have removed from yourself and those that belonged to the other person and throw them on to the fire that burns at the entrance of the door that you came in through. Leave the crystal room in peace and with the freedom to continue your life.

With the busy lives that so many people lead, it is very easy to forget about protecting oneself. One way to remedy this is by getting into the habit of protecting yourself as soon as you wake in the morning and ensuring that the method used will be potent for 24 hours. I feel that this is of great importance, especially for those working in the public sector, and those who travel on crowded buses and trains. It is also advantageous to protect your car before setting out on a journey. I have proved for myself on more than one occasion that this works. When I step into the car I ask the angels, archangels and the Christ light to guide and protect it during the course of the day. I then visualise a circle of cosmic light surrounding the car.

I personally feel that the time has come when we must learn to become the masters of our own energies by knowing how to protect them and how to cleanse the energies in our surrounding space with the strong vibrant energies of light. This will enable us to mix with all types of people and be involved in the multitudinous situations of life. To prove the efficacy of these protection techniques and any others that you might read about, observe over a period of months the changes they make in your life.

CHAPTER 9

CONTACT HEALING WITH PRANIC ENERGY

EVERY TRADITIONAL culture sees life as a vast limitless energy force that resides in physical objects for a certain length of time. The Greeks named it *pneuma*, the ancient Indians called it *prana*, the Japanese named it *Qi*, to the Chinese it was known as *chi* and the Native Americans referred to it as 'the flow of the spirit'. When an individual's way of life affects the amount of life force they are able to absorb, illness manifests in the physical body.

Many practices have evolved which aim to strengthen a person's life force and these were used by many religious orders as the basis for their spiritual life. The discovery of the Dead Sea scrolls revealed that the Essenes, a Jewish sect living an ascetic, communal way of life in desert locations, formally trained people in the laying on of hands and it is believed that some members of their community possessed a great gift for channelling energy in this way. Cave paintings of the healing practices of the Native Americans also depict the laying on of hands and this healing touch has been and still is used throughout Asia. One of the aims of yoga is to utilise *prana* to strengthen, vitalise and keep the body in optimum health and one of the ways this is achieved is through control of the breath. Taoist philosophy, acupuncture and the martial arts are all based on developing a mature understanding and utilisation of this underlying life force for health, wisdom and personal power.

At the present time, scientists are researching this ancient wisdom by examining the effects of hands-on healing on animals, children and adults. Their studies have shown that people receiving contact healing have increased alpha brain waves, which induce relaxation, diminish stress, improve respiration, hormonal balance and bowel function, lower blood cholesterol levels and strengthen the immune system.

In 1961, the *International Journal of Parapsychology* published an article by Dr Bernard Grad from the McGill University in Montreal under the title of 'The Influence of an Unorthodox Method of Wound Healing in Mice'. This article stated that the wounds of laboratory mice treated with contact healing healed faster than similar wounds on mice treated in the conventional way. The article continued by showing evidence that plants grew faster, stronger and produced more chlorophyll when they were given the healing touch. I personally have seen the effect that contact healing has on both plants and animals.

One of the pioneers and practitioners of Therapeutic Touch, Dr Dolores Krieger, reported in 1979 in an article, 'Therapeutic Touch: Searching for Evidence of Physiological Change' in the *American Journal of Nursing* that haemoglobin increased in patients receiving this treatment. In 1987, Dr Janet Quinn reported in the same journal under the title 'One Nurse's Evolution as Healer' that amongst subjects receiving Therapeutic Touch there was an enhanced ratio between CD4 cells, the helper T-cells that direct the immune response against an antigen (a substance which causes the formation of antibodies) and CD8 cells (cells that shut off the immune system). These findings are of particular importance for those suffering HIV and AIDS, because these people suffer from a diminishing number of CD4 cells and an increase in CD8 cells. This causes a decline in the immune system and a failure in its response to cancer cells. (See also Dr Krieger's book, *Living the Therapeutic Touch: Healing as a Lifestyle*, Dodd, Mead & Co., 1987.)

Another pioneer in this field is Professor Robert Becker, an orthopaedic surgeon and formerly a professor at Upstate Medical Center New York. He has shown that the auric field around a person contains a unique intelligence that controls the growth, development and health of cells and tissue. Along with other scientists he has proved that the human body is animated by a complex web of electrical energy and he has worked with a variety of techniques, including contact healing, to enhance this. He has found that when this energy is enhanced, the immune, endocrine and nervous systems are strengthened and the body's own healing power is raised. In his book *Cross Currents: The Perils of Electropollution, the Promise of Electromedicine* (Jeremy P. Taroher, 1990) he talks about how the body uses electrical control systems to regulate many basic functions and how the flow of these electrical currents produces externally measurable magnetic fields. He postulates that the healer's gift is an ability to use their own electrical control systems to produce electromagnetic energy fields that interact with those of the patient. Professor Becker concludes, 'The interaction should be one of those that restores balance in the internal forces or that reinforces the electrical systems so that the body returns to a normal condition.'

I personally believe that the complex web that Professor Becker speaks about are the nadis contained in the etheric layer of the aura and that the electrical current is the *prana* which flows through these. When, as colour practitioners, we work with contact healing we are working in the same way but are using the specific frequencies which constitute *prana*, namely colour.

BECOMING SENSITIVE TO COLOUR AND *PRANA*

To work with colour contact healing, we need to become sensitive to the vibrational energies of colour and the electrical current, *prana*. We need to learn how to channel this energy through ourselves to the patient and how to revitalise ourselves in the process. The sensitivity gained through such practices is extremely beneficial when feeling and working with the aura in healing. The exercises given below are designed to help you heighten your sensitivity to pranic energy and colour and to increase your own energy reserve. To do this, practice must be on a regular basis.

Sensitising the Hands to *Prana*

Sitting quietly, place the palms of both hands together. Feel where they make contact and take note of any sensations passed from one to the other. Gently move them approximately 8cm apart and visualise as white light the pranic energy which is building up in the space between both hands. This energy is generally felt as a slight pressure that tries to push the hands away from each other. As the pranic energy increases, slowly move your hands apart until you are able to hold between them a large ball of white light.

When you feel that this ball has reached its maximum size, transfer it to any part of your body where you are experiencing discomfort or disease by placing your hands at your chosen spot and visualising the white ball of pranic light being absorbed into the pain or discomfort. This exercise can be repeated until the discomfort starts to ease.

Working with the Breath and Visualisation

Pranic Visualisation Sitting

Sitting comfortably on a chair with the soles of both your feet on the floor and your hands on your knees, release any tension in your physical body. With a relaxed body and straight spine, start this exercise by taking a few normal breaths, allowing your concentration to be centred in the breath. Slowly start to inhale and exhale more deeply. With each inhalation, visualise an intense white light entering your nose and flowing down into your solar plexus. Continue to visualise this until your solar plexus becomes a ball of glowing energy.

Now place your fingertips on your solar plexus. Continue to breathe *prana* into your solar plexus but with each exhalation see the intense white light pass from your solar plexus through your fingertips and into your hands.

When your hands have become radiant with light, transfer them to any part of your body where there is pain or disharmony. Slowly exhaling, visualise the white pranic light flowing from your fingertips into the chosen part of your body. Now return your fingertips to your solar plexus and repeat until the pain or discomfort has subsided.

Pranic Visualisation Standing

Standing with your feet slightly apart and your hands by your sides, exhale deeply to rid the lungs of as much stale air as possible. As you take a deep and slow inhalation start to raise your arms, visualising a tiny ball of pranic energy starting to form in your solar plexus. Continue the slow deep inhalation until the palms of your hands meet over the top of your head. Both arms should be kept straight. Retain the breath for a count of five while concentrating on the white ball of light forming in your solar plexus. Now begin a slow exhalation bringing your arms back to your sides. Continue to repeat the above process until the ball of white pranic light is large enough to fill your solar plexus.

Now with your arms by your sides and your body relaxed, visualise this ball of light sending out rays of pranic energy to every part of your body. Try to feel the extent to which you have been energised.

Adding Colour

Colour can be added to both the above exercises. In the first exercise, when your solar plexus has become a glowing ball of energy, visualise the colour you need permeating this light. You should visualise red, orange and yellow coming from the earth, through the soles of your feet to your solar plexus, green horizontally entering the heart chakra and radiating down to the solar plexus and turquoise, blue, indigo, violet and magenta coming down into your solar plexus through the top of your head. Next place your fingers on to your solar plexus and when your hands are filled with your chosen colour, transfer it to any part of your body where you feel this colour is needed.

If you wish to add colour to the second exercise, work with the above instructions until your solar plexus is filled with white light. Keeping your arms by your sides and your body relaxed, visualise your chosen colour entering the ball of white light until it glows like a coloured sun and radiates its rays of colour to every part of your body.

ALTERNATE NOSTRIL BREATHING

Everywhere in the external world we encounter manifestations of the positive–negative principle and a certain balance must be maintained between these two principles. Likewise a constant balance must be contained in the constant interplay of positive–negative pranic current in the two main nadis. These are the *pingala* (positive) and the *ida* (negative). Both these nadis originate from the base chakra and terminate at the brow chakra. *En route* from the base chakra they circulate in opposite directions round the chakras that lie between their points of origin and termination. A breathing exercise which helps to balance this positive–negative pranic current is alternate nostril breathing, or *sukh pavak*.

Sukh pavak

Sitting comfortably on a chair with the soles of both feet on the floor, check that your spine is straight and your body relaxed. Keeping your left hand on your knee, place your right thumb against your right nostril: your index and middle finger together on your forehead, between and just above your eyebrows, and your ring and little finger against your left nostril. Pressing the right nostril closed with the thumb, inhale through the left nostril to a count of six. Press the left nostril closed with your ring and little finger and exhale to the count of six through the right nostril. Keeping the left nostril closed, inhale through the right nostril for a count of six and then press the right nostril closed with your thumb, open the left nostril and exhale through it to a count of six. Without pausing, inhale through your left nostril to a count of six. This completes one round.

Without pausing perform 10 more rounds.

When you have completed these, place your hands on your knees and breathe normally. Reflect for a few moments on how you are feeling.

Alternate nostril breathing not only balances the positive and negative flow of *prana* through the *ida* and *pingala* nadis but also rejuvenates the nervous system.

When you are familiar with the sequence of this exercise, visualise inhaling the brilliant white light of *prana* and with each exhalation see this energy permeating the network of nadis constituting the etheric body.

WORKING WITH A PARTNER

This exercise is designed to help you to channel energy into another person. In the initial stages only work with channelling white light, but when you feel confident you can ask your partner which colour they feel attracted to and using the same technique, you can work with channelling this colour.

Channelling Energy into Others

Sit comfortably on a chair, with the soles of both feet on the floor, facing your partner, who has adopted the same sitting position. Your partner's left hand should rest on their left knee with the palm facing towards the ceiling and their right hand should rest on their right knee with the palm facing down. Place your right hand on top of your partner's left hand and your left hand under their right hand. Take a few slow even breaths to calm your mind and relax your body.

When you feel ready to begin, bring your concentration to the crown of your head and visualise a beam of white light there. On your next inhalation bring this beam of light down into your heart chakra, where it becomes permeated with unconditional love. On your next exhalation, take this light from your heart centre down your right arm and into the chakra in the palm of your right hand. From here visualise it being transferred into the left hand of your partner, where it travels up their left arm, through their heart chakra, down their right arm to the chakra in their right hand. From this chakra it passes into your left hand, up your left arm and back to your heart chakra to complete a circuit of pranic energy.

With each inhalation continue to breathe white light into your heart chakra and with each exhalation visualise this travelling round the circuit you have just created.

Practise this exercise for 10 to 15 minutes. Now break the circuit by removing your hands from your partner's and placing them on your own knees. Discuss with each other your experiences and any difficulties you may have encountered.

When you become proficient at this exercise, you can work in the same way with the colour your partner feels the need for. When working with colour bring red-orange and yellow through your feet to the heart chakra. Green enters the heart chakra horizontally and the colours above green enter the heart through the head.

LEARNING TO FEEL COLOUR

If we have chosen to work with the vibrational energies of colour, it is important that we learn how to feel and to recognise each colour's energy.

Feeling Colour

The simplest way of doing this is to get yourself pieces of material dyed with the 12 tertiary colours (or you may wish to dye the material yourself, which will give you the exact shade of the colour required).

When you have gathered your material, sit down in a place which is quiet and warm and place the colours around you. Taking each colour in turn, place it on the palm of your left hand then hold the palm of your right hand approximately 7cm above the piece of material. Closing your eyes, try to feel through your right hand the energy of the colour you are holding. In between feeling each colour, place your hands on to the floor and dedicate any energy remaining on them from the last colour to be laid to the earth. If this is not done the vibrational energy from each colour will accumulate on your hand, making it very difficult to differentiate between each colour's vibrational energy. Make notes of any sensations felt with each colour.

Another way of working with this exercise is using flowers or crystals in as many of the 12 colours as possible. The colours found in flowers and crystals are more vibrant and this makes it easier to experience their energy.

CHAPTER 10

CONTACT COLOUR HEALING: A STEP-BY-STEP TREATMENT

CONTACT COLOUR healing is the incorporation of colour into Therapeutic Touch, a healing art derived from the ancient practice of laying-on of hands. Therapeutic Touch involves the channelling of life energy or *prana* through the hands of the practitioner to the patient to release blockages of energy, to balance disharmonious rhythms and aid the recipient to assimilate the *prana* being channelled. Any practitioner wishing to work in this way must develop a sensitivity to the subtle energy or aura which surrounds and interpenetrates the physical body, and learn to focus their mind. The best way of perfecting the latter is through meditation.

When working with therapeutic touch you are channelling all the colours constituting *prana*. In contact colour healing the vibrational energies of specific colours are being channelled to the organs and systems of the physical body alongside the aura. The colours channelled are either the general or treatment colours.

The step-by-step treatment given in this chapter has evolved from the techniques taught at the Maitreya School of Healing and is one of the methods being taught by The Oracle School of Colour. It is a method which might interest those practising Therapeutic Touch or Reiki.

The therapy room where treatment is administered should be clean, tidy and have a peaceful, relaxing atmosphere. The colours used to decorate this room are important and ideally should contain a lot of blue or pale violet. The room should not be cluttered, containing only the things needed by the practitioner for giving treatment. These would include for example a therapy couch, two chairs, maybe a small desk, a filing cabinet for patients' records and the instruments used for treatment.

When the patient arrives, the first step is to take down their personal details, their medical history and their present state of health. A spine chart is made and interpreted for them (see Chapter 6) and the treatment procedure is described so that they are aware of what is happening. There is nothing less conducive to relaxation than lying on a couch wondering what is going to happen to you. The patient is then asked to remove their shoes, to loosen any constricting clothing and to lie on the therapy table, which should be covered with couch roll for hygienic purposes. This should be renewed for each patient. A pillow, also covered with couch roll, should be placed under the patient's head and one should be placed under their knees if they suffer back problems. A thin white blanket can be used to cover them to make sure that they do not get cold during treatment. This may happen because their metabolic rate slows down as their body relaxes.

As you prepare to begin the treatment, take a moment to remind yourself that you are only the channel through which the healing energies of colour flow. Ask that you may be a good and clear channel and that you may be guided by divine power. Your approach should be humble and confident as you help a fellow soul on its way. Before you begin, make sure that you have protected yourself from picking up any negative energies that may be present and bear in mind the following contra-indications.

Caution when Working with Specific Diseases

Glaucoma

This disease is caused by the intraocular pressure being so high that it actually damages the nerve fibres in the retina and optic nerve. If a patient attends complaining of severe eye pain they should be referred to their doctor immediately.

Underactive thyroid

If the thyroid is underactive, it is not producing enough of the hormone thyroxine and is usually treated with thyroxine tablets. These tablets are also given when the thyroid gland has been partially or totally removed. If a patient is taking thyroxine and still has the whole or part of their thyroid gland, it is important that they are monitored by their doctor throughout the colour treatment because colour therapy can activate this gland to produce more thyroxine, so the amount being taken orally may have to be reduced.

Cancer

Tumours of the prostate, uterus, thyroid and some breast cancers are treated with hormone therapy. This is used to change the hormonal balance in the body by reducing, increasing or blocking the action of a certain hormone. Some tumours are affected by the hormone levels in the body and changing this level may prevent or destroy such tumours. For patients receiving this treatment it is not advisable to work with the endocrine system or the chakras because this could counteract the medical treatment being prescribed.

Diabetes

If a patient is taking insulin it is important for them to monitor themselves after treatment. Colour therapy could activate the islets of Langerhans to produce more insulin and this would make it necessary for the patient to reduce their intake.

Contra-indications for Colour Therapy

Red

This colour should not be given to those suffering asthma, high blood pressure, hypertension, hyperactivity, insomnia, heart disease or those who are bleeding. It is not a good colour to use with the eyes, especially if the person is suffering eye strain.

Orange

This is a colour which stimulates the appetite, making it harmful for people with eating disorders. It should also be used with discretion on people with addictions.

Yellow

This colour stimulates mental activity and is not a good colour for those suffering mental exhaustion. Exposure to this colour for any length of time could make one feel 'spaced out'.

Blue

Blue as a main colour is not recommended for people suffering depression or seasonal affective disorder because it can aggravate the condition, but it can be given as the complementary colour to orange. It is also not recommended for those with low blood pressure.

STEP 1

The first step is to clear the aura of stagnant energy. Always start with the patient's head because this is the seat of the soul, the most sacred part of the body temple and it deserves special attention. Place your hands approximately 5cm above the patient's head in the etheric part of their aura and slowly work across their head and face and down their body, feeling for the presence of stagnant energy with your hands. This is usually felt as an excess

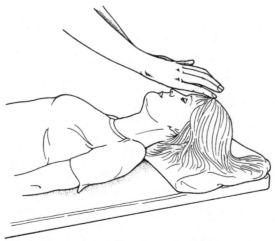

Step 1 – Clearing the aura

of heat or cold or as a tingling sensation. It is dispersed by channelling the colour of pearl or iridescent white through your hands for a few seconds. When you have completed this part of the treatment, take a few seconds to reflect on your findings.

After you have cleansed the aura, the next step is to channel colour into the body. The colours given in this step-by-step treatment are the general colours, the colours which each part of the body vibrates to naturally, but if the patient is suffering a specific disease you would treat the parts of the body affected with the colour and complementary colour recommended for that disease.

When channelling colour, visualise it entering your body and flowing to your heart chakra, where it is infused with unconditional love, before flowing down your arms and into your hands. Red, orange and yellow come from the earth and enter through your feet, green enters horizontally into your heart centre and turquoise, blue, indigo, violet and magenta enter your body through the crown of your head.

When working with colour visualise the colours displayed in nature because plants are very responsive to the sun and all plants exhibit some degree of phototropism. This sensitivity to the sun means that plants produce the very refined colours suited to healing application.

The way in which all the colour vibrations exhibited through the plant kingdom blend together, united by an all-pervasive undertone of green, provides a living demonstration of harmony. This is the harmony which we seek to bring to those coming for treatment. When working with these flower colours, we strive to transmit the healing essence of their colours to the patient. This 'essence' is the unique, pure, intense healing beauty of each flower, which draws forth the beauty of the patient. That beauty is the healer within.

STEP 2

Starting with the patient's head, place your hands over the crown and visualise the colour displayed by violet flowers coming through your hands, entering their crown chakra and flowing into their brain and pineal gland.

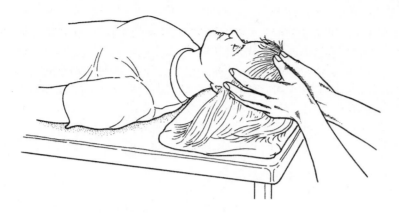

Step 2 – Working with the crown of the head

The Brain

The brain is contained and protected within the rigid bony case of the skull. It is divided into three main parts: the cerebral hemispheres responsible for controlling functions such as speech, memory and intelligence; the cerebellum, which controls co-ordination movement and balance; and the brain stem, which merges into the top of the spinal cord and maintains the vital functions of the body, such as breathing and circulation. Nerve signals travelling through the spinal cord link the brain with the rest of the body. Special attention is given to this part of the body for those suffering from epilepsy, cerebral palsy, headaches, migraine, multiple sclerosis and trigeminal neuralgia.

The Pineal Gland

The pineal gland is situated on the upper part of the mid brain and is a small reddish structure approximately 10mm in length. This gland's melatonin secretion is affected by light and in some animals plays a part in hibernation and in controlling sexual activity. In humans it controls the rhythms of the body throughout the 24-hour day, induces sleep and influences our moods.

STEP 3

Removing your hands from their crown, place them beneath the patient's head with your fingers positioned on the alta major chakra. Visualise the golden colour of the trumpets of King Alfred daffodils and buttercups flowing into this chakra and down the spinal cord to energise the whole of the nervous system.

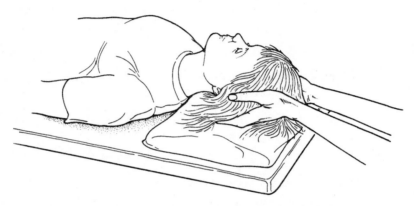

Step 3 – Treating the alta major chakra

The Spinal Cord

The brain and the spinal cord together are known as the central nervous system. The spinal cord is a soft column of nerve tissue continuous with the lower part of the brain and enclosed in the bony vertebral column. This column stretches from the base of the skull to the bottom of the buttocks and consists of 33 small bones called vertebrae. These vertebrae are linked by strong ligaments and have flexible discs composed of a jelly-like substance encapsulated in a tough fibrous outer covering.

Stemming from the spinal cord are 31 pairs of peripheral nerves which pass through narrow side channels in the vertebral column to the head and body. The peripheral nerves that run to the body are named after the four regions of the spine from which they branch. These are the cervical, thoracic, lumbar and sacral regions. There are two types of peripheral nerves. The first type are the sensory nerves which convey nerve impulses from sensory organs to the brain and the second type are the motor nerves which carry messages from the brain to the various muscles of the body.

Apart from the peripheral nerves there are 12 pairs of cranial nerves which run from the underside of the brain to various organs and parts of the body. Some of the more important cranial nerves carry information from the main sense organs to the brain where it is co-ordinated and interpreted.

STEP 4

Carefully and gently remove your hands from beneath the patient's head and place the first two fingers of each hand on to the brow chakra. This is located between the eyebrows and works with the pituitary gland. Channel a deep indigo into this centre.

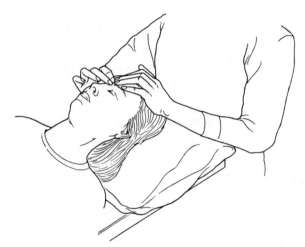

Step 4 – Treating the brow chakra

The Pituitary Gland

The pituitary gland is approximately the size of a peanut, sits just beneath the brain and is the most important gland in the body. It consists of an anterior and posterior lobe. The anterior lobe produces six hormones responsible for growth, for activating the breasts to produce milk, for stimulating the thyroid, the adrenals, the ovaries and the testes. The posterior lobe produces hormones which act on the kidneys and stimulate the uterine contractions in childbirth. This chakra and the pituitary gland are important points for treatment in those suffering hormonal imbalances.

STEP 5

When you have finished treating the brow chakra run your fingers across the forehead and down either side of the head to the minor chakra situated in the small indentation at the base of each ear. First visualise a lighter shade of indigo entering these points then treat both ears with this colour by covering them with your hands.

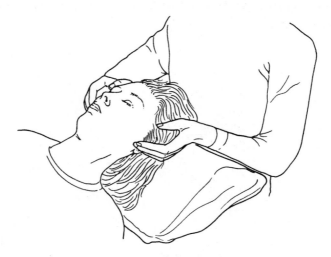

Step 5 – Treating the ears

The Ears

As well as enabling us to hear, our ears are important as organs of balance. Each ear consists of three parts: the outer ear, the part we see, the middle ear containing the eardrum and the inner ear. When sound waves fall on the eardrum they cause it to vibrate. These vibrations are then passed to the fluid in the inner ear, causing it in turn to vibrate. These vibrations stimulate nerve endings which carry impulses to the brain.

STEP 6

Still working with indigo, treat the patient's eyes by gently covering them with the palms of your hands, making sure that no pressure is exerted.

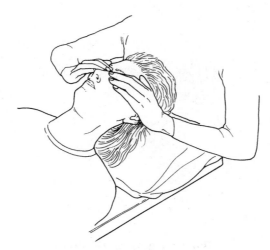

Step 6 – Treating the eyes

The Eyes

The eyes, as explained in an earlier chapter, are very important organs not just for vision but for allowing the body to assimilate both the light and colour which are so important for our well-being.

STEP 7

Removing your hands from the eyes, place them over the cheeks of the face to treat the sinuses with indigo.

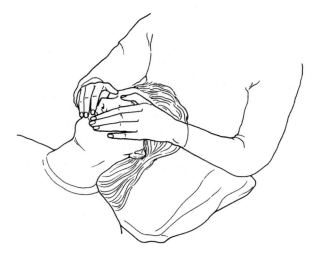

Step 7 – Treating the sinuses

The Sinuses

These are air-filled cavities and their function is to reduce the weight of the head and give resonance to the voice. They are lined with a membrane which secretes mucus which drains into the nose. Sinusitis usually develops from a cold or bacterial infection but the sinuses can become infected as a complication of the swelling of the mucous membrane associated with allergic rhinitis.

STEP 8

Taking your hands away from the face, place the first two fingers of both hands on to the throat chakra. This is found in the notch in the throat lying between the two clavicle bones and is linked with the thyroid and parathyroid glands. Visualise the blue of delphiniums flowing through your fingers into this centre. When you have finished treating this chakra, wrap your hands around the front and sides of the neck to treat the larynx, trachea, vocal cords and neck muscles with the same colour.

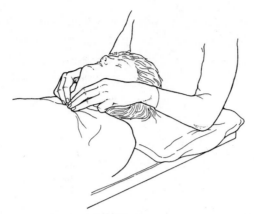

Step 8 – Treating the throat chakra and neck

The Thyroid Gland

The thyroid gland is situated in the lower neck and consists of two lobes, one on each side of the trachea, joined by a thin strand of thyroid tissue. It produces the hormone thyroxine which controls the rate at which chemical reactions occur in the body. An essential constituent of thyroxine is the chemical iodine.

The Parathyroids

Embedded in each of the four corners of the thyroid gland is a parathyroid gland which is approximately the size of a pea. These produce the parathyroid hormone which, together with vitamin D, controls the level of calcium in the blood.

STEP 9

When you have treated the neck, place the palm of each hand midway along each clavicle bone and visualise blue flowing from your palm chakras into the minor chakras situated at this point on each clavicle bone. These points are important in people suffering from neck and shoulder tension.

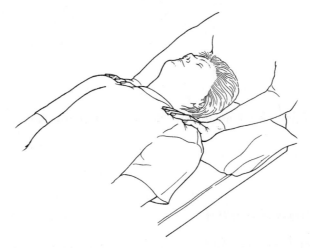

Step 9 – Treating the minor chakras of the clavicle bones

STEP 10

Still keeping your hands in contact with the patient, move your position to the patient's left side. Starting with your hands positioned at their left shoulder, channel a light blue into their shoulder, arm, hand and fingers as you slowly run your hands down these parts of their body.

When you have completed treating the left arm and hand, move to the right side of the couch to treat the right arm in the same way. If the person is suffering any problems with their shoulder, elbow, wrist or finger joints, cup these between both hands and channel the colour and complementary colour recommended for the complaint.

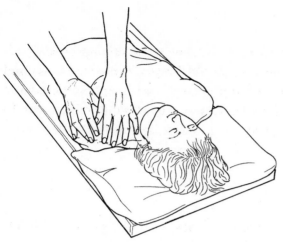

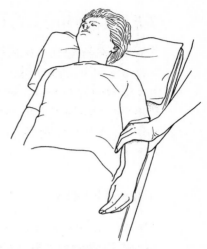

Step 10a – Treating the shoulders and arms   Step 10b – Treating the elbow joint

STEP 11

After treating the arms, place the first two fingers of both hands on to the heart chakra. This is located slightly to the right of the physical heart, which it influences alongside the thymus gland.

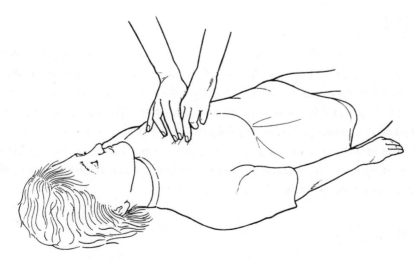

Step 11 – Treating the heart chakra

The Thymus Gland

The thymus gland was given its name by Galen in the second century AD because of its resemblance to a bunch of thyme flowers. It has two lobes and lies in the upper part of the chest. It consists largely of lymphoid tissue and plays a part in the formation of lymphocytes, a type of white blood cell. In infancy these lymphocytes are coded to recognise and protect the body's tissues.

The Heart

The heart lies in the chest between the two lungs with two thirds to the left of the breastbone and the remaining third to the right. It is encased within a strong fibrous bag known as the pericardium.

The heart is a hollow muscular pump with four cavities, each provided at its outlet with a valve. Its main function is to maintain the circulation of the blood. The right side of the heart pumps blood to the lungs, where waste gases are removed and oxygen added. Freshly oxygenated blood returns to the left side of the heart, from which it is pumped to all organs and tissues.

STEP 12

If you are working with a female patient place your hands gently over her breasts and channel a light green into this area. Then, without moving your hands or changing the colour, imagine the etheric part of your hands passing through the patient's body to encase and treat their lungs. If you are treating a male patient you would treat the lungs immediately after treating the heart chakra. I have found that quite a number of people have an accumulation of stagnant energy around this area which I believe is due to the amount of pollution in the air we breathe.

The Breasts

The female breasts overlie the second to sixth ribs on the front of the chest and are made up of fat, supporting tissue and glandular tissue which is responsible for producing milk following childbirth. On the surface of each breast is a central pink disc called the areola which surrounds the nipple. Around each nipple are 12 to 20 compartments. These open on to the tip of the nipple via its own duct, through which the milk flows. The milk secretion is due largely to the hormone prolactin with contributions from progesterone and oestrogen.

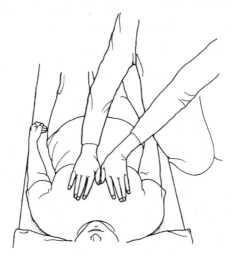

Step 12 – Treating the breasts and lungs

The Lungs

The two lungs are situated in the chest on either side of the heart. In young children these are a rose pink but in adults they tend to turn a slatey grey due to deposits of inhaled dust and pollution. Each lung is encased in a membrane, the pleura or pleural membrane. The right lung is slightly larger than the left lung and is divided into three lobes by two deep fissures. The left lung is divided into two lobes by one fissure. The texture of the lungs is very elastic and each lung is composed of tiny air sacs called alveoli. When we inhale, the cavity of the thorax is enlarged to make room for the lungs to expand into. When we exhale, the thorax returns to its former size as the air is expelled from the lungs.

STEP 13

When you have finished treating the lungs, move your hands down to the solar plexus chakra. This is situated just above the navel and is linked with the pancreas, especially the islets of Langerhans (see below). With the first two fingers of both hands placed on this point, visualise the yellow of gorse bloom being channelled into it through your fingers.

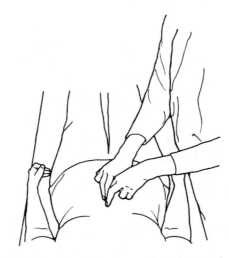

Step 13 – Treating the solar plexus chakra

The Pancreas

The pancreas is situated at the back of the abdomen behind the lower part of the stomach. It is composed of tubes of columnar cells and scattered throughout these are collections of cells known as the islets of Langerhans. These cells produce insulin. The main function of the pancreas is the formation of pancreatic juices which contain the enzymes needed to digest proteins, convert starchy foods and to break up fats. The insulin produced by the islets of Langerhans is secreted directly into the bloodstream to utilise sugars.

STEP 14

Still working with yellow, move your hands to the right side of the body and place them side by side, just below the ribcage. This is where the liver and gall bladder are situated. If you feel the patient's liver is toxic, change the colour you are channelling to lime green.

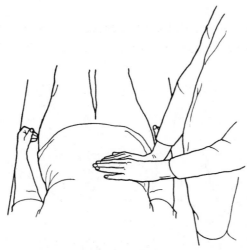

Step 14 – Treating the liver and gall bladder

The Liver

The liver is a solid, dark brown organ and one of the largest glands in the body. It is triangular in shape and divided into four lobes. The largest of these is the right lobe and the gall bladder is attached on the underside of this. The liver is often described as a vast chemical factory and the heat produced by the chemical changes taking place in it forms an important contribution to the warming of the physical body. Amongst its many chemical activities are the production of bile and the manufacture of enzymes, cholesterol, complex proteins, vitamin A and blood coagulation factors. It neutralises toxic substances from the small intestine and aids in the metabolism of protein, fat and carbohydrates.

The Gall Bladder

The gall bladder is a sac approximately 8cm in length. Its function is to store and concentrate the bile secreted by the liver that helps break down fatty foods. When bile is needed for this, it is passed through the bile duct and into the small intestine by muscle contraction.

STEP 15

After treating the liver and gall bladder, place both hands horizontally across the body, under the ribcage, to treat the stomach with yellow.

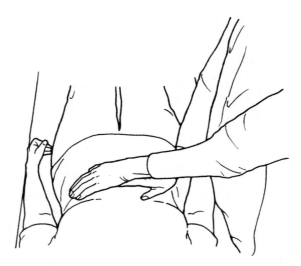

Step 15 – Treating the stomach and pancreas

The Stomach

The stomach is situated mainly on the left side of the body and it acts as a food reservoir and food processor. Food enters the stomach through the oesophageal sphincter and once inside powerful muscles in the stomach wall crush the food, which is further broken down by hydrochloric acid and enzymes made in the stomach lining. When the food has been processed it passes out of the stomach through the pyloric sphincter, into the duodenum.

STEP 16

From the stomach, move your hands to the left side of the body and place them side by side just under the ribcage to treat the spleen with gold.

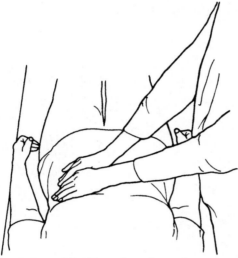

Step 16 – Treating the spleen

The Spleen

The spleen is situated behind the stomach on the left side of the abdomen. It is a soft, vascular, plum-coloured organ with a smooth surface. Its function is to produce lymphocytes and to act as a reservoir for red blood cells. Old red and white corpuscles and platelets are broken up by the spleen and from this process bilirubin is produced and conveyed to the liver and iron which is used in the bone marrow for the production of new red blood cells.

STEP 17

To treat the kidneys and adrenal glands place your left hand on the right side of the patient's body and your right hand on their left side diagonally across the waistline. Visualise your etheric hands extending into the body to treat both these organs with a daffodil yellow.

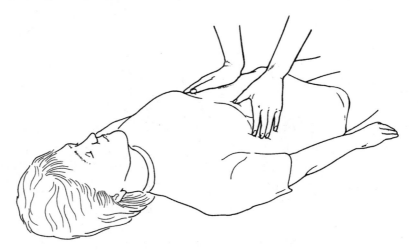

Step 17 – Treating the kidneys and adrenal glands

The Adrenal Glands

The adrenal glands are two organs approximately 5cm in length and sit one on the top of each kidney. Each adrenal gland consists of the medulla (the inner layer) and the cortex (the outer layer). The medulla, stimulated by the brain, produces adrenaline and noradrenaline, two hormones which play an important part in controlling blood pressure and heart rate. The cortex produces three types of steroid hormones which are responsible for chemical balance in the body, the conversion of carbohydrates into glycogen in the liver and the production of the male and female sex hormones (these sex hormones are also produced by the ovaries and the testes).

The Kidneys

The kidneys are situated diagonally across the waistline on either side of the spinal column. The left kidney is slightly longer and narrower and lies marginally higher in the abdomen than the right. Both kidneys are surrounded by fat which cushions and supports them. Each consists of the cortex (the outer layer) and the medulla (the inner part). When blood from the renal artery reaches the cortex, it passes through minute globular structures which filter off liquid containing nutrients and waste products from the blood. The filtered liquid passes from these globular structures into the medulla along a long thin tubule surrounded by blood vessels which reabsorb the nutrients from the liquid. The remaining liquid continues along the tubule into the ureter and is collected in the bladder as urine.

STEP 18

From treating the kidneys and adrenal glands move your hands down to the lower abdomen to treat the sacral chakra, situated just below the navel, with the orange seen in the petals of marigolds. This chakra is linked with the adrenal glands described in Step 17.

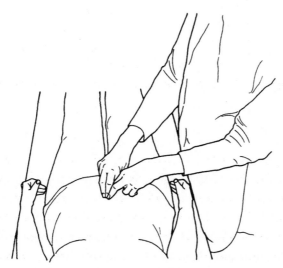

Step 18 – Treating the sacral chakra

STEP 19

From the sacral chakra move both of your hands down to the lower part of the abdomen to treat the bladder and the small intestine with orange. This is done by placing the heel of both hands just above the pubic bone with your thumbs together and the remaining fingers splayed across the abdomen.

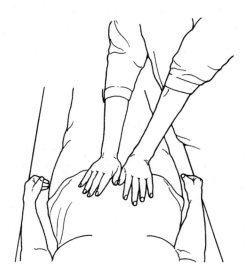

Step 19 – Treating the bladder and small intestine

The Bladder

The urinary bladder is situated in the pelvis in front of the last part of the bowel and has elastic flexible walls. It is able to contain approximately half a litre of urine which is passed from the kidneys, down the ureter tubes and into the bladder. Each ureter tube is linked to the bladder by a valve which prevents a back flow of urine when the bladder contracts. When the bladder is full the sphincter muscle relaxes, allowing the bladder to contract and discharge urine down the urethra.

The Small Intestine

The small intestine is a tube approximately 7m in length suspended in loops in the abdominal cavity. It is divided into three parts: the duodenum, into which the ducts from the liver and pancreas open, the jejunum and the ileum, which at its lower end opens into the large intestine. Like the stomach, the small intestine is constantly in motion controlled automatically by a network of nerves, pushing the food along its length by peristaltic waves of contractions of the muscles in its walls. The semi-digested food from the stomach passes into the small intestine where the secretion of enzymes from the intestinal walls, bile from the gall bladder and pancreatic juice from the pancreas further the digestive process. Once the food molecules are small enough, they pass through the thin lining of the intestine into the bloodstream and then on to the liver for storage and distribution.

STEP 20

Following the small intestine, the colon or large intestine is treated in two sections with orange. To treat the first section, which is the ascending and transverse colon, stand on the left side of the patient and place your left hand, fingers facing towards the head, along the right side of their abdomen and your right hand horizontally across their body, just on the waistline. To treat the descending and sigmoid colon, place your right hand, with fingers pointing towards the head, along the left side of the abdomen and your left hand, with its heel placed against the heel of the right hand, sloping down to the pubic bone.

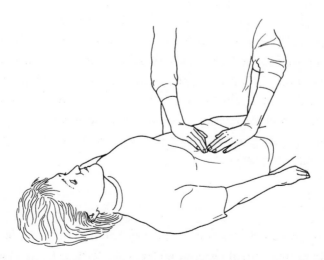

Step 20a – Treating the ascending and transverse colon

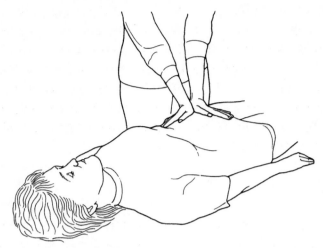

Step 20b – Treating the descending and sigmoid colon

The Colon

The colon or large intestine is approximately 1.5m long and consists of two main sections, the colon and the rectum. The small intestine opens into the colon through a pouch like chamber called the caecum. From here the colon runs up the right side of the body (the ascending colon), across and under the ribcage (the transverse colon), down the left side of the abdomen (the descending colon). The descending colon sinks into the pelvis, where it becomes the sigmoid colon. The last part of the large intestine is the rectum, which is a tube about 12cm in length leading to the anus. Through the membranous wall of the colon, fluids and various mineral salts are absorbed from its contents into the bloodstream. Any indigestible solids are compacted and propelled towards the rectum, where they are stored as faecal matter ready for release through the anus.

STEP 21

When you have finished treating the colon, place your hands horizontally across the pelvis, just above the pubic bone, to treat with orange the uterus and ovaries in a female and the prostate gland in a male.

The Ovaries and Fallopian Tubes

The two ovaries and uterus lie in the lower part of the abdomen and are the main organs of female reproduction. The ovaries lie on either side of the uterus and each is connected to the uterus by a Fallopian tube. The ovaries are shaped like almonds and are whitish in colour. Their main functions are to produce ova, to prepare the uterus for pregnancy through their hormonal secretions of oestrogen and progesterone and to transform a girl's body into that of a woman at puberty. The ovaries become active during puberty through stimulation by the gonadotrophins, the hormones secreted by the pituitary gland.

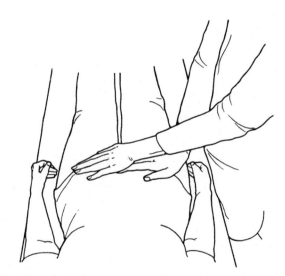

Step 21 – Treating the uterus and ovaries or prostate gland

The Uterus

The uterus is a hollow organ suspended by ligaments in the cavity of the pelvis. It is approximately 8cm in length with thick muscular walls. The lower end of the uterus is prolonged into the rounded cervix which is about 2cm long and protrudes into the vagina. The uterus is where a fertilised ovum becomes embedded and develops into a baby. If pregnancy does not occur, the lining of the uterus breaks down and is discarded through the menstrual flow.

The Prostate Gland

The prostate gland surrounds the urethra at the point where it leaves the bladder and comprises a cluster of small glands. These glands secrete an alkaline fluid during ejaculation and this is a constituent of semen.

STEP 22

Placing your hands just above the pubis, first visualise a clear red being channelled through your hand chakra to treat the base chakra and then lighten this colour to treat the testes in a male.

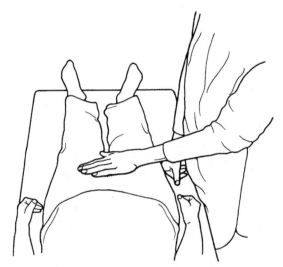

Step 22 – Treating the base chakra and testes

The Testes

The testes are linked to the base chakra and are the male reproductive organs. They are suspended outside the body in a scrotum. Each testicle consists of a gland that produces sperm and testosterone, and a long tightly coiled tube called the epididymis. Sperm manufactured in the testes is passed into the epididymis to mature before being propelled into the vas deferens and then into the seminal vesicles, where it is mixed with the seminal fluid produced there.

STEP 23

Having completed treatment on the lower abdomen, the next step is to treat the spine with a golden yellow. Starting at the patient's neck, place your hands vertically down the centre of the body and slowly slide your hands down their body to the pubis to encompass the whole spine. At each stage, visualise your etheric hands passing through the body to make contact with the spine. (The spine is described earlier – see pages 82–98 and Plate section).

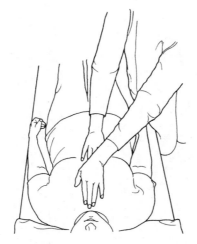

Step 23a – Treating the upper spine

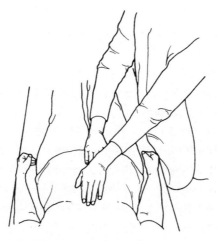

Step 23b – Treating the lower spine

STEP 24

When you have treated the spine, place both hands at the top of the right leg and working with red, move your hands in a criss-cross movement down the leg and across the foot. Repeat this action on the left leg and foot. If the patient is suffering problems with their hip, knee or ankle joints, place your hands around these joints and channel the appropriate colour, with its complementary colour, for the complaint.

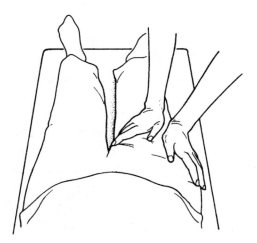
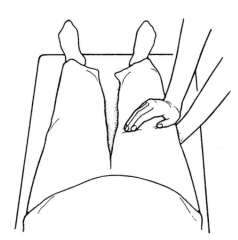

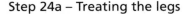

Step 24a – Treating the legs   Step 24b – Treating the knee joint

STEP 25

This last step of the treatment is administering the overall colour, found from the spine chart, through both the patient's feet. The feet are a mirror image of the whole body, therefore administering the overall colour through them is equivalent to administering it to the whole body.

Placing your left hand on the patient's left foot and your right hand on their right foot, visualise the overall colour flowing through your hands and into their feet. Continue to do this for about three minutes before changing to visualising the complementary colour, which is administered for the same length of time.

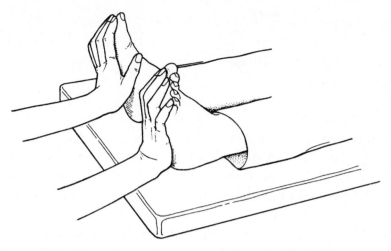

Step 25 – Administering the overall colour through the soles of the feet

When you have finished the treatment, cover the patient with a blanket and leave them to relax for a few moments while you go and wash your hands. You should wash your hands to just past your wrists. This breaks every connection with any disharmonies encountered during the healing session and stops you from passing these on to another patient or absorbing them yourself. The temperature of the water is not important, but the action of the water running over your hands is.

After washing your hands, return to your patient and gently rouse them. Invite any questions that they wish to ask before instructing them how to work with the overall colour between treatments. These methods are explained in the next chapter.

Finally make your patient a further appointment if you think this is necessary, before bidding them farewell.

THE CANDLE TECHNIQUE

This is a specialised technique used at the end of a healing session, to help cleanse and strengthen sensitive, frail and emotionally weak people. It is nearly always applied to the back, very rarely to the front of the body. For this procedure you will need a lighted nightlight placed in a small dish.

When the colour contact session is complete, gently rouse your patient and ask them to turn over so that they are lying face downwards with their arms about 5cm away from their body and the palms of their hands facing towards the ceiling (see opposite).

Step A

Commence treatment by holding the candle approximately 16cm above the patient's head then start to move the candle down the left side of their head, along their neck and shoulder and down the outer side of their arm to their hand. Over the palm of their hand make the sign of the equi-limbed cross in the circle.

Continue by moving the candle up the inner side of their arm and down the left side of their body to their foot. Again, on the sole of their foot make the sign of the cross in the circle.

From their foot take the candle up the inside of their left leg and down the inside of their right leg to the sole of their right foot where the sign of the cross and the circle is traced.

Proceed up the right side of their body, down the inside of their right arm to the palm of their right hand where you trace the sign of the cross and the circle before continuing up the outside of their right arm, across their right shoulder, up their neck and the right side of their head to the point where you started.

Step B

From this point weave the candle from left to right over their body until you reach their feet. Sweep around their feet and return to their head, this time weaving the candle from right to left.

Step C

When you reach the crown of their head, take the candle down the centre of their body to the base of their spine. As you move back up their spine to the crown, make the sign of the cross and the circle over each of the major chakras to seal and protect these.

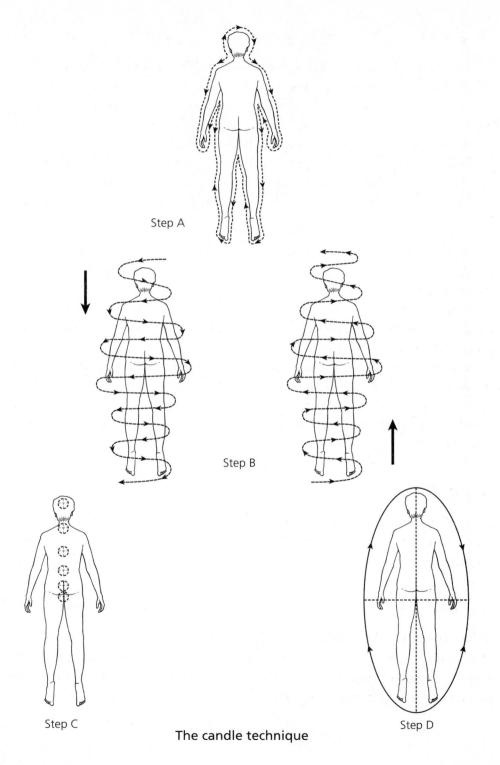

Step A

Step B

Step C

Step D

The candle technique

Step D

After sealing the crown chakra take the candle back down the centre of the patient's body to their feet. From here bring it back to their waist, where it is moved horizontally to the left to approximately 5cm beyond their body, then moved the same distance to the right of their body. Returning to the centre of their body, bring the flame back to the crown.

This movement has placed the person into a cross of light. To finish walk all round their body with the flame to place them in a protective circle of light. Blow out the candle and leave your patient to rest for a few minutes.

CHAPTER 11

WAYS OF WORKING WITH COLOUR

THE COLOUR THERAPY INSTRUMENT

Contact colour healing, though of great benefit, can prove difficult for practitioners who lack colour sensitivity, who have difficulty in keeping their mind focused or for those who do not wish to come into physical contact with their patient. On the other hand, there are patients who feel that they have not received a treatment unless they see the colours they are being treated with. For those people who find contact healing difficult and for patients who psychologically gain more from seeing the colours, the colour therapy instrument is ideal.

I personally feel that the colour instrument and contact healing both have something special to offer. In contact healing, working with our intuition and with our higher self allows the exact shade of the colour needed to be channelled through us. On many occasions I have felt a different colour from the one I was visualising coming through my hands. When this happens, it serves to remind us that each individual is unique and may therefore require a different colour from the one normally given for their condition. Other advantages with contact healing are being able to locate and clear any areas in the aura where there is stagnant energy, the benefits gained from treating the separate parts of the body with either their general or treatment colours, and the work that can be done to balance the chakras. With the colour therapy instrument we are only able to work with the overall colour and its complementary colour, but its advantages lie in its ability to show the patient the colours they are receiving and for them to absorb these colours through their eyes and skin.

The colour therapy instrument comprises two glass-fronted wooden boxes placed one on top of the other on an adjustable stand. Both boxes are connected to a controller which controls the treatment time and the change sequences between treatment colour and complementary colour. Both boxes are fitted with a lamp and have slots into which the stained-glass filters slide. The top compartment houses the overall colour and the lower compartment the complementary colour (see below).

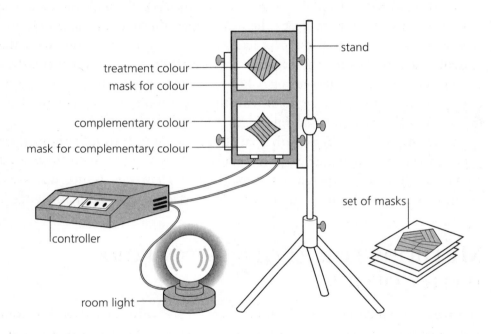

The colour therapy instrument

When a patient attends for treatment with the colour therapy instrument their personal details and medical history are recorded. A spine chart is made and interpreted for them. They are then asked to go to the bathroom to remove all coloured clothing, because this will act as a filter changing the colour they are being treated with, and to put on the white treatment gown provided.

While they are doing this, the coloured filters determined by the spine chart are mounted in the instrument and the room darkened except for a small working light which is switched off at the commencement of the treatment. Ideally a blackout blind should be used to give maximum darkness because light dilutes colour, so the darker the room, the stronger the colours being transmitted.

When the patient is ready, they are seated on a comfortable chair, the working light is switched off and the colour therapy instrument switched on. The sequence of changes from colour to complementary colour lasts for just under 20 minutes and for the colour to be absorbed through the eyes it is important that the patient keeps their eyes open throughout the procedure. It is equally important for the practitioner to stay in the room with the patient and this calls for the need for the practitioner to protect themselves from receiving the colour (see pages 119–30). Staying with the patient can be both a comfort and provide them with the opportunity to express any feelings or thoughts that arise during the treatment.

At the end of the treatment the patient is encouraged to talk about their experiences before being given instructions on how to work with the overall colour during the following six days. Longer than this is not advisable because as the condition of the patient changes so do the colours they need.

METHODS FOR PATIENTS TO WORK WITH COLOUR

The ways in which patients themselves can work with their overall colour and if need be the complementary colour are many, but one way which is not recommended is the use of coloured light. Bathing a person in coloured light is a very powerful treatment and best left to a qualified colour practitioner. There are patients who believe that extending the recommended treatment time quickens the healing process. This is not always true and could prove dangerous if coloured light were being used.

Solarising Placebo Tablets

I have found the easiest and most powerful way for a patient to work with their colour and complementary colour is with placebo tablets solarised by the practitioner with the required colours. The patient benefits from this method psychologically as well as physically, because taking tablets to cure disease is what most people are conditioned into believing works. Also, taking a tablet is less time-consuming than working with other methods and is therefore more likely to be remembered.

To solarise placebos you will need some sac lac tablets, obtainable from most large homoeopathic pharmacies, a small wooden box with two compartments painted white and a set of stained-glass filters to fit over each compartment. The tablets are then placed into the compartments of the box and the appropriate filters placed on top. This is then left on a windowsill for approximately one hour on a bright sunny day and up to four hours on a dull grey day. The solarised tablets must then be placed in black-labelled pots to prevent them losing their colour potency.

The patient is given six tablets of each colour and instructed to take one tablet solarised with the overall colour half an hour before breakfast and one tablet solarised with the complementary colour half an hour before lunch for six days.

It is very important to stress the importance of taking the complementary colour. When I was experimenting on myself with this method, I solarised and took two blue tablets half an hour before breakfast and two blue tablets half an hour before lunch. By the time evening came I couldn't stop crying and wondered why. Then light dawned and I realised that I had not taken the complementary colour of orange. After remedying this, I began to feel really well and full of vitality.

Since prescribing these tablets to patients, I have seen some truly remarkable results. One lady was suffering acute depression related to problems at home. I gave her tablets solarised with orange and blue and instructed her to take these for six days. At the end of this time she returned for another treatment and said she was amazed at how quickly the depression lifted after starting the treatment and this new sense of well-being enabled her to look at and start to resolve the underlying cause of her problem.

To a patient suffering infected sinuses, I gave red and green tablets. When he returned for his next treatment he reported that the condition had initially got worse but after two days on the treatment the sinuses discharged a lot of greenish mucus and by the end of the week the condition had almost cleared.

For practitioners choosing to work with this method, I would recommend getting either some medium-sized black pots or white jars that can be painted with black glass paint, labelling each of these with one of the colours used and then storing solarised tablets in them ready for use when needed. When these are given to a patient they also need to be stored in tiny black pots or small black envelopes. The latter can be easily made from black paper, obtainable at most good art shops.

Lunarising Tablets

A method developed from solarising tablets is lunarising them. This idea came after seeing quite a few patients suffering menstrual and hormonal problems. The tablets are prepared in the same way as for solarising but instead of being placed in sunlight they are 'lunarised' with the light of the full moon.

Because the opportunities for doing this are less frequent, it is advisable to lunarise as many colours as possible when the moon is full and the sky clear. These can then be stored in the same way as solarised sac lac but it is important that the label differentiates them from the solarised tablets.

Visualising Colour

Visualising colour is very powerful if it is worked with regularly. This takes time, and if the patient is willing to spend this time working with themselves they will greatly benefit. When working in this way I always instruct the patient to work with the colours displayed through flowers or minerals and suggest that they find either or both of these in the colour they need. These colours are living and vibrant and have a great healing capacity. I also recommend that they choose the same time each day to practise because this creates a good habit that is easy to follow. The following is an example of a visualisation that you might like to work with.

Working with Red and Green

For this a red tulip is needed. Place this in a vase where you can see it comfortably. Look at its shape and colour and then, when you feel ready, close your eyes and visualise the head of the tulip increasing in size until it is large enough for you to walk inside and sit or lie at its centre.

When you are comfortably positioned inside the tulip, imagine the sun shining through its petals, creating shafts of soft red light which bathe you from head to foot. Try to feel the effect that this has upon you physically, emotionally and mentally.

After approximately 15 minutes, walk out of the tulip on to one of its long and slender green leaves. Pause here for a moment to absorb this complementary colour through your feet, before walking down the tulip's leaf back to where you are sitting. Visualise the tulip returning to its normal size before gently opening your eyes.

You might ask the patient to find a different red flower to work with each day or to create a different visualisation which they write down and bring with them on their next visit.

Meditation with Colour

This method is best suited to those who have some experience with meditation. When meditating it is important to find a quiet place where you will not be disturbed. The ideal time is early morning after a good night's sleep. This eliminates the temptation to fall asleep. The sitting position adopted should be one that is comfortable and allows the spine to be straight. If you choose to sit on a chair, make sure that both feet are placed on the floor with your hands, palms downwards, on your knees. With your eyes closed, start your meditation with five minutes of rhythmic breathing. This helps to quieten the mind and relax the body. At the end of your meditation it is important to close down the major chakras. These are your doors to higher consciousness which open during meditation. The simplest way of closing them down is to visualise each chakra as an open flower. Starting with the crown chakra, visualise each flower closing back to a bud.

Meditation with Indigo

When your mind has become quiet and your body relaxed, imagine that you are sitting in front of a giant quartz crystal. Standing up, walk round the crystal to find the entrance to its inner chamber.

When you have located this door, open it and walk through into a room whose walls, ceiling and floor are constructed from crystal. On the floor lies a deep indigo thick-piled carpet upon which are scattered indigo and white cushions. Hanging from the ceiling are spirals of indigo glass balls which fill the room with wide shafts of indigo light. Walk around this room to see what else there is to discover before gathering some of the cushions to place under your head and beneath your knees, if you suffer back problems.

When you are lying comfortably with your cushions in position, take note of your body bathed in the indigo light flooding the room. If you listen carefully you will hear the gentle tones being sounded by the crystal. Everything in the universe is singing and their collective sounds are known as the music of the spheres but these gentle undulating harmonies are inaudible to most people.

Become aware of your physical body to experience how this colour induces a wonderful state of peace and relaxation to both your body and mind and how it creates space for you to be yourself.

When you feel refreshed and re-energised, stand up and walk out through the door of the crystal. Start to become conscious of your physical body sitting on the chair. Then visualise the crystal returning to its normal size. Now open your eyes and feel revitalised for the day that lies before you.

Breathing in Colour

Breathing in colour requires time but it is a relatively easy exercise to do because the breath is always with us, we do not have to go out and find it. It is advisable to practise by an open window in the morning because the intake of *prana* revitalises the body and could lead to insomnia if practised late at night.

There are many breathing techniques but the simplest is the rhythmic breath. With this the inhalation is the same length as the exhalation. How long you choose to make the breath will depend upon your lung capacity. Try starting with a count of three for both the in breath and the out breath. If you find this relatively simple, increase the count to five or to seven. When practising always return to normal breathing if you become dizzy or find that you are out of breath.

Breathing in Violet and Yellow

When you are ready, start this exercise by taking a few rhythmic breaths to find your lung capacity. When you feel comfortable with this, visualise with every inhalation a shaft of violet light entering the top of your head and pouring down through your body to your feet. With every exhalation visualise a shaft of yellow light entering the soles of your feet and rising up through your body to the crown of your head.

Another way is to work just with the violet for the first five minutes and then change the colour to yellow.

Try both of these methods and see which one works for you.

Using coloured material as a filter

To work with this you will need to get a full length piece of silk or cotton material in the required colours. The reason for using silk or cotton is because these are natural fabrics which do not restrict the aura. Synthetic fabrics do restrict the aura, preventing its natural expansion and contraction, and this can be detrimental to health. The best source of silk or cotton is Indian fabric shops. These normally supply a vast range of colours at nominal prices. I see no advantage in buying expensive material for this practice; it serves no purpose. Indian shops also supply material which is made from a percentage of silk and cotton and this is cheaper than pure silk. If you find a shop which has a good, cheap supply of material, it is beneficial to buy a length of material in all the colours to keep in your therapy room. You will find these useful both for demonstration purposes and for your own work.

Working with a Length of Orange Material

When working with coloured material, you need to remove all coloured clothes because these will also act as a filter and distort the colour that you are trying to assimilate into your body.

Find a place which is light, warm and quiet. Lie down with a pillow beneath your head and cover yourself from your neck to your feet with the length of orange material. If you find music relaxing, have your favourite piece playing softly in the background. Now close your eyes and relax for 20 minutes.

If you find it helpful, repeat the exercise later in the day using a piece of blue silk. Red, orange and yellow are stimulating colours and should be worked with in the morning.

Another way of using material as a filter is to wear clothes in the colour you need. Again, you must wear white underneath to prevent other colours being filtered. Sometimes I am asked if the colour can be worn in underwear. The answer to this is yes, but you would have to wear white on top and I do not think it would look very elegant to wear a red bra underneath a white blouse!

I would recommend colour practitioners to work with the above methods. This will give them the insight and experience needed to choose the exercise best suited for their patient as well as increasing their own sensitivity to colour.

CHAPTER 12

ABSENT HEALING

Absent healing is a powerful and effective form of healing that is used with people who are too ill to attend a clinic or who live too far away. One question frequently asked is, 'If absent healing is so effective, why can't all sick people be treated in this way?' I feel there are many reasons why; the most important lies in the fact that absent healing is unable to give the warmth, love and physical contact that a patient receives throughout a colour therapy treatment. Another advantage of contact healing is the patient's involvement in the healing process. The effort made to attend the clinic is a step made by the patient to help themselves and this effort stimulates the healing process. Attending a clinic for treatment gives the opportunity to discuss problems, fears and worries with the practitioner and this is a step towards resolving them. For some, the therapist is the only person they feel able to discuss their personal life with, and this is done trusting that any information imparted will not be discussed outside the therapy room.

GAINING PERMISSION

To give absent healing we first have to receive permission from the sick person, because this form of healing can create great changes in a person's life and they may not wish for these changes. They could also become frightened or worried if they felt changes occurring within themselves that they had no explanation for. There are those who would argue that a person will block the healing energy if they don't wish to receive it. This may be true for the physically strong, but it is not the case for those made physically weak through ill health.

I know an elderly lady who was admitted to hospital after suffering a heart attack. When I visited her in hospital I asked if she would like me to send her healing. Looking very distressed, she declined this offer because she was aware that a great deal of healing energy was being sent to her which she was finding very difficult to handle. She said that she could not ask for this to be stopped because she had no idea who was sending it. I know from personal experience how powerful this energy can be. When I was ill, if I had not first been asked if I would like to receive absent healing, I would certainly have been alarmed at the movement of energy this caused in my body.

I personally feel that giving absent healing without the person's consent is to interfere with their free will and this is wrong. The only exception to this rule is when we visually lift a person into the light of the universe and ask that they be given what is right for them at that moment in time: 'Thy will not mine be done.'

GAINING INFORMATION

There are several ways of performing absent colour healing, but for all of these techniques information on the patient and the disease they are suffering is required. We need to know if we are treating a child, baby or adult and if, for example, they are suffering from cancer, which part of the body this is affecting. All this information helps us to select the appropriate treatment.

If possible, tell the patient when healing will be sent and suggest that they find a quiet relaxing place at that time to concentrate on and become more receptive to the energy that is being transmitted. As well as being beneficial, this encourages them to partake in their healing process.

ABSENT COLOUR HEALING USING VISUALISATION

This technique requires us to visualise the person we are working with and to project beams of coloured light from our brow chakra to individual parts of their physical body. To become proficient at this requires practice in colour projection and concentration. Before working with this method, take time to practise the exercise given below.

Colour Projection

Sitting comfortably and quietly, start this exercise by concentrating for a few minutes on your inhalation and exhalation. This will help to relax and quieten your mind. Continue by imagining a beam of white light entering your right and left eye and travelling to your hypothalamus, which sends it to your pineal gland and crown chakra, your pituitary gland and brow chakra and your carotid glands and alta major chakra. As these centres become infused with light, visualise three light triangles forming in your head. The first of these is formed with the crown, brow and alta major chakras, the second with the pineal, pituitary and carotid glands and the third with the right and left eye and the pineal gland. Now imagine in front of you, approximately 30cm from your body, the black outline of a rose, a chrysanthemum, a daffodil, a bluebell, an iris and a pansy on a white background. Bringing your concentration to your brow chakra, project from this place a beam of red light to colour the petals of the rose. Change the colour to orange to colour the chrysanthemum, then yellow for the daffodil, green to colour the stems and leaves of the flowers, blue for the bluebell, indigo for the iris and violet for the pansy. When you have completed this you might like to try working with colour tints to add shading to the different coloured petals.

As you become more experienced at working in this way, try visualising in black and white a country or seaside scene and then paint it by using the same method.

Working with Visualisation for Absent Healing

If possible, set aside the same time each day for this work. Find a place in your home where it is warm and where you will not be disturbed. If you are able to keep this space for your spiritual and healing work, over a period of time it will become imbued with a very vibrant and uplifting energy which will help you. If you find it helpful place crystals and flowers around you and maybe a set of coloured scarves to help you focus on the healing colours. You will need also a white candle in a holder and some matches.

Before starting your healing session light the candle and dedicate its light to those who have asked for healing, asking at the same time that you may be a good channel for that energy and for protection for both yourself and your patients. Adopt a comfortable sitting position, either on a chair or on the floor, but whichever posture you adopt, make sure that your spine is kept straight. Practise rhythmic breathing for a few minutes to quieten your mind and relax your body.

Visualisation (1)

When you feel ready to start your work, visualise your patient lying in a beautiful garden filled with colour from the flowers and trees that grow there and surrounded by light and warmth from the sun.

Keeping your mind focused on the patient, visualise a narrow beam of violet light radiating from your brow centre into the patient's crown chakra. After a few seconds change the colour to indigo to treat their face and brow chakra and then to blue to treat their throat chakra, the neck, both arms and hands. From their hands bring your focus back to their chest and use green to treat all the organs and muscles which lie in their chest cavity. If you feel that the person lacks love and/or is suffering emotional pain and trauma, first project violet into their heart chakra followed by rose pink. These two colours serve to mend a broken heart before filling it with unconditional love. Changing the colour to yellow, visualise this treating their solar plexus chakra, stomach, liver, gall bladder and pancreas. After treating these organs change the colour to gold and apply it to their spleen to create energy for their physical body. Now focus your attention on their lower abdomen and visualise a beam of orange light from your brow chakra entering first their sacral chakra and then the organs contained in this part of their body. Lastly change the colour to red to treat their base chakra, both legs and both feet.

At the end of the treatment surround the person in an orb of protective white light and visualise them in a relaxed and peaceful state. Extinguish the candle before washing your hands in cold water to break all contact.

The above visualisation uses only the general colours but in a sick person, these would be replaced with the treatment colour and its complementary colour in the parts of their body suffering disease. When working with this method, instead of visualising the person lying in a garden you can visualise them lying on a couch in a therapy room or sitting against a tree in woodland or in a forest. Sitting against the trunk of a tree brings one within the aura of the tree, allowing the absorption of its energy and strength. This is a beneficial exercise for practitioners after giving treatment but it is important to thank and bless the tree before leaving it.

Visualisation (2)

Sitting quietly, visualise a circular rose garden encased within evergreen shrubs, with a fountain playing at its centre. The roses are in full bloom, filling the air with their delicate perfume and displaying the many shades of red, white, yellow and peach. The garden is filled with sunlight, flooding the fountain and filling each tiny droplet of water with the warmth of its healing rays. Scattered around the garden are comfortable reclining chairs.

Visualise those who have requested healing entering the garden through the wooden gate set amongst the evergreen shrubs and selecting one of the chairs to sit on. Sitting and absorbing the spectacle of colour surrounding them and breathing in the delicately perfumed air releases the strain and tension frequently seen on the faces of those suffering ill health. As you watch them relax, ask the universal light to give them understanding of their present disease and the wisdom to find the path to wholeness.

After a short period of rest, see them rising from their chairs and walking towards the fountain. At the fountain's edge they first place their hands into the water to test its warmth then immerse themselves in it. As they stand beneath the cascading water, visualise the vibrant healing light encapsulated within each tiny droplet being released into the areas of their body where there is disease or disharmony. Visualise these areas as a dark grey mist which slowly dissolves in the presence of this liquid light.

At the appropriate time, see each person step back from the fountain and with an air of joy and rejuvenation, walk back to and out of the gate.

ABSENT HEALING USING THE SPINE CHART

Using this method, the spine chart is made either from the handwriting on the letter sent requesting treatment or, if the request was made by telephone, from the patient's photograph requested during the telephone conversation or from a spine chart sent to them for signature.

When making the chart, work with a lighted candle for the protection of both yourself and your patient and as a reminder that all healing energy comes from the universe through you. If after giving treatment, either with the person present or with absent healing, you feel drained of energy, then you are doing something wrong. This usually happens because you are giving of your own energy but it can also happen if you are feeling unwell or working from your ego. If this continues, it will be you who ends up being ill. All good practitioners find that they are energised at the end of a treatment by the energy that they have been channelling.

When the chart has been made the unbridged vertebrae are treated for approximately 15 seconds with the colour and the complementary colour attributed to them. This is done either by channelling the colour through your middle finger or with a colour therapy torch (see below). This torch has a white plastic head fitted with a quartz crystal to amplify the vibrational energy of the stained-glass filters which fit inside it. The unbalanced chakras on the chart are treated with the appropriate colours in the same way. A full interpretation of the chart is then written up, in layman's terms, and sent to the patient with suggestions on how they can work with the overall colour.

If you feel that the patient would benefit more from taking sac lac, then send them six tablets potentised with the overall colour shown on the chart and six potentised with the complementary colour. These should be placed

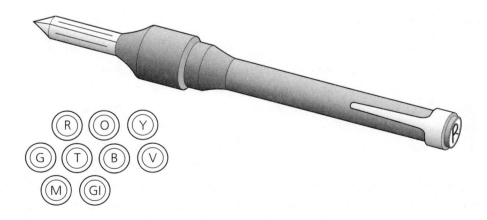

The colour therapy torch

in two separate, small, black, labelled envelopes with instructions on how they are to be taken. I have found that psychologically a patient benefits more from being given something to take than from being given visualisation or colour breathing exercises. Benefiting psychologically aids the healing process.

Another way of administering the colour and complementary colour is through the colour therapy instrument. To do this a photograph of the patient is needed. This is pinned to a white cloth which is secured to the back of a chair. The room is darkened and the appropriate colours relayed through this instrument are projected on to the photograph for just under 20 minutes.

USING GEOMETRIC FORM IN HEALING

For this method you will require a shallow box of sand, some small birthday cake candles in all the colours, a photograph of the person asking for healing and a box of matches. You will then need to select one of the geometric forms given on page 189 to work with. Again, this can be done with dowsing or you may intuitively know which shape to use.

Geometric form with colour is used by some healers because each form contains its own vibrational energy which enhances the colours used. The forms most generally used are the triangle, the square, the equi-limbed cross, the pentagram, the six- and seven-pointed star and the circle.

The Triangle

In ancient times the triangle was regarded as a symbol of light. When placed with its tip pointing upwards it represents the sun and symbolises life, fire and the masculine energy. Placed in the reverse position it connects with the moon, water and the feminine energy. The triangle is aligned with the number three and in Christianity this represents the Trinity and the body, mind and spirit of man. In Hinduism the upward and downward triangles are the Shakta and the Shakti, the linga and yoni or Shiva and his Shakti. When this symbol is used in absent healing it amplifies the healing force and aids the colour by helping it to work on all aspects of the person. It therefore benefits those who are inwardly searching to find themselves or the cause of the complaint they are suffering.

The Square

The square represents the solidity of the earth and totality through the depiction of the four elements earth, fire, air and water in its four sides. It contains the qualities of honesty, integrity and morality and helps people who are trying to find these virtues within themselves. In Hinduism the square is the archetype and pattern of order in the universe, the standard and the perfect measure for man. When used with absent healing it helps to provide security, protection and wholeness and balances the four elements found in each person. It is also beneficial in helping to ground a person by 'keeping their feet on the ground'.

The Equi-Limbed Cross

This cross symbolises the four corners of the Earth, the four elements and the four states of man. The horizontal line is the earthly, rational, passive and feminine and the vertical is the spiritual, intellectual, active and masculine. The two lines together represent our dualism which ultimately leads to polarity and wholeness. Each person has a right and left hemisphere to the brain, they contain both the masculine and feminine energy, require the heat and activity of the sun and the passive, coolness of the moon. In working with polarity all these aspects are balanced to create wholeness.

In Indian philosophy polarity is likened to a pendulum on a clock along which all individuals are positioned. When the pendulum swings to the right, feelings of well-being and joy are experienced, but when it swings back to the left, these turn to depression and unwellness. The pendulum returns to the right, bringing emotions of love and harmony, but then returns to the left, changing these emotions to ill-humour and irritability. To work with polarity, we must climb up the pendulum to the point where it is fixed to the clock. Here there is no movement and this symbolises that we have reached that state of integration and wholeness.

In healing the equi-limbed cross is used for those who need to look at their imbalances and work towards alignment and harmony.

The Pentagram

The five points of the pentagram represent earth, water, fire, air and spirit, and the five senses of sight, hearing, touch, taste and smell. Its shape symbolises the figure of a man with legs and arms outstretched. The Pythagoreans believed this to be a symbol of health and knowledge. In Christianity it symbolises the five wounds of Christ and in Hinduism it is seen to be Prakriti, the feminine power of creation and manifestation, the universal mother, the quintessence of the natural universe. This shape is linked with the angels of healing, the Cherubims, and is used in absent healing when we wish to invoke these beings to help in our healing work. It also adds strength to the energies of the colours being used and works with the person's spirituality.

Six-pointed Star

This is formed from two interlocking triangles. In its two-dimensional form it represents the Star of David and in its three-dimensional form is known as the star tetrahedron. It is the union of opposites, the upper triangle is usually white and masculine and the lower one black and feminine. It signifies the perfect balance of complementary forces and the androgynous nature of the deity. In absent healing this symbol works with a person's duality as well as strengthening and providing protection for them.

Seven-pointed Star

All stars reflect light and when used as symbols of healing they send light and hope into the darkest corners of a person's life. The seven-pointed star talks about completeness, security, safety and rest. In absent healing it is symbolically used for a person who has to make major changes in their life and for balancing and aligning the seven major chakras. It is the symbol that is always used with children.

The Circle

The circle talks of timelessness because it has no beginning and no end and spacelessness because it has no above or below. It gives one a sense of secu-

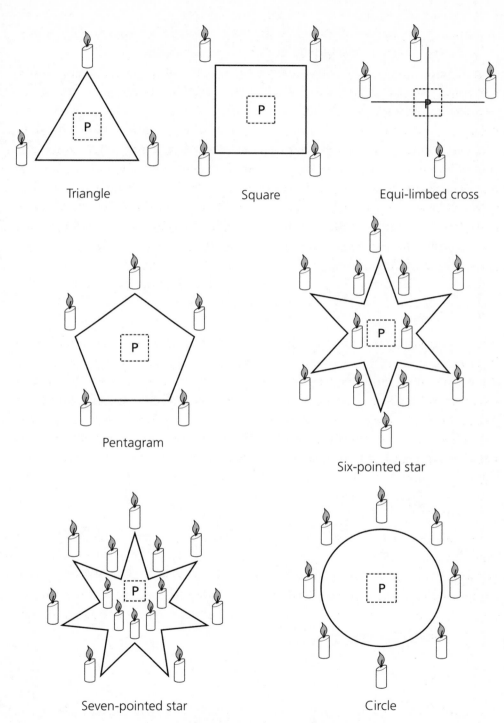

Triangle

Square

Equi-limbed cross

Pentagram

Six-pointed star

Seven-pointed star

Circle

Candle layout for absent healing

rity and anything enacted within a circle is protected. The psychologist C. G. Jung sees the circle as the psyche and the true self.

In absent healing this symbol is used with the vulnerable and with those who need protection and security while they are working to solve the problems facing them.

When working with geometric form in absent healing first find the overall colour either through dowsing or by making a spine chart. I personally would recommend a spine chart because this can give important information on the person's well-being. When the overall colour has been determined, use tiny birthday candles in this colour, to create the geometric form you have chosen to work with in the sand box. Into the centre of this form place the photograph of the person you are working with, then light the candles. Dedicate the light from these to be sent to the person for healing. Leave the sand box in a safe place for the candles to burn out.

The Power of Prayer

If you feel you would like to work with the power of prayer I would suggest that you keep a list of those people who have asked you for healing. Keep this in the place where you do your absent healing work. If you practise meditation on a regular basis, either at the beginning or the end of your practice visualise the people who have asked for your help being lifted into a cloud of white light and ask that each individual receive what is right for them. In doing this, you have placed them into the healing hands of the universal light.

CHAPTER 13

DEATH AND DYING

THE BEST FORM of healing for a person may in fact be their physical death. Those of you who are working or training as complementary therapists will encounter death, in all its various stages, more frequently than the average person. For this reason it is of vital importance that you feel comfortable in its presence and have no fear of it. Theoretically accepting the concept that healing sometimes takes the form of death and that death liberates the soul from the prison of form is the first step in accepting and losing any fear you may hold.

In some Eastern countries the birth of a child is a time of sorrow because the soul has lost its freedom by incarnating into a human form, but death is a time of great rejoicing because the soul has regained its freedom. When we stand free of all resistance to and fear of death, our healing work takes on a deeper power for, as expressed in the 'seed thoughts' of the Maitreya School of Colour: 'The healer celebrates life and fears neither birth nor death nor any change in form.'

If we ask ourselves what death is, a simple answer would be a transition from one form into a more subtle form. Orthodox science usually describes death as a closing down of all physical functions resulting in an ending of life. Esoteric science, which dates back further than orthodox science, takes a different perspective. It speaks of a 'sea of life' in which death and birth are simply stages of its existence, passages of transition in a larger concept of cosmic wholeness. This concept is beautifully demonstrated by nature: a tree comes into bud, the bud opens into a leaf which brings new energy and life to the tree. After a while the leaf changes colour, then fades and falls to the ground. Here it rots and becomes reintegrated with the soil and with Mother Earth. Meanwhile the tree lies dormant, resting until spring when the whole process begins anew.

Each of us experiences a mini death daily. Every night during sleep we leave our physical body and function in the astral world. The only difference between this and death is our connection to the physical body by the magnetic thread, or current of energy, along which the lifeform streams, which is preserved intact and constitutes the path of the return to the body. In death, this life thread is broken, preventing the conscious entity's return to the dense body.

During the night our astral activities are numerous and varied. A soul which is not yet spiritually awake will hover around its physical body awaiting the call to return on the awakening of its physical vehicle. The souls of spiritually-orientated people frequently meet loved ones already in spirit, carry out specific tasks for which they have been chosen and receive insights which help them with projects they are working with on Earth. Unfortunately most of the night's work is forgotten on waking. One technique which can be employed to bring those experiences back to waking consciousness is to keep by your bedside a notepad and pencil. This is used to recall your dreams immediately upon waking, before they fade into obscurity. The next step is learning to decipher which of your dreams were astral travels and which were the release of emotions from the unconscious mind.

WORKING WITH THE DYING

One way of experiencing death in its many forms is to work for a minimum of one year in palliative care. I myself did this for two years and found the experience invaluable. The palliative care centre where I worked as a complementary practitioner had several wards plus a day care centre attached to it, enabling me to work with those who were very near to death, those in remission and those whose life expectancy ranged over several months.

Prior to doing this, I enrolled for a weekend course on cancer for complementary practitioners at the Lynda Jackson Centre which is attached to Mount Vernon Hospital. This hospital has a large cancer unit which employs complementary practitioners from a variety of disciplines. It was explained during the course of this weekend that when a person is first diagnosed with an incurable disease, their first response is shock, an inability to take in the information received, withdrawal and denial of the situation. Following this comes fear – fear of the outcome; of the reaction of friends and family, and the mutilation of their body through possible surgery. Then comes the uncertainty about treatment and how successful it will be in dealing with the disease, coupled with worry about the side-effects of some of the drugs given. The final stage is acceptance of the situation.

When we as practitioners work with the dying this knowledge is of prime importance in helping us to understand how these people feel and how we can help them through each stage of their crisis. Another important aspect is having the understanding and ability to accept and unconditionally love them as a human being no matter what condition their body is in or how they initially react to us after receiving the news that they are terminally ill. Also, if we as practitioners are frightened to discuss death or ourselves fear this stage of life then we need to confront this issue within ourselves and resolve it before working with such people. The dying are frequently very sensitive to the feelings of others and will pick up on any fear or negativity surrounding those who are trying to help them.

There were several special occasions in my work with the dying that I can recall. The first was working with a man in palliative care the day before his death from motor neurone disease. The only part of his body that he was able to move were his eyes. As I worked with him, I was filled with wonder and a tremendous feeling of peace from the warmth and unconditional love radiating from his eyes. I felt as though his soul, which was about to leave his physical body, was speaking with great love and strength to those in attendance.

The second vivid memory that I have was again treating a patient just two days before he died. He was unable to speak but could manage to sit in a chair. I sat gently massaging his hands, working on the various reflex points. After finishing work on his right hand and before treating his left hand, he gently took hold of my hand and started to massage it. This was, I felt, his way of saying thank you.

Another occasion was when I was treating a patient at my home for terminal cancer. She had undergone surgery and was receiving a course of chemotherapy. On her second visit to me, she entered the therapy room and without warning removed the wig she was wearing, threw it on to the floor then looked for my reaction. Fortunately, seeing a bald head as a result of chemotherapy was not a new experience for me and therefore I had no reaction. Noting this, she settled down for her treatment. What was interesting was that on subsequent visits, she kept her wig on.

When attending the dying it is important to remember to refrain from talking if the person is unconscious. Usually, even in the face of unconsciousness, the patient's faculty of hearing is still present, enabling them to be aware of all that is happening around them. Idle chatter can prevent the departing soul from making a smooth transition to the spiritual world. The burning of orange candles in the room and the playing of soft, gentle music will help the soul. In America, the Chalice Midwives, an order which works with the dying, sit at the head of the dying person and intone certain sounds to help the soul disconnect from its physical vehicle. You might also like to work with prayer and visualisation. Visualise the soul of the dying one peacefully leaving their body and walking into the light of God. You might also see them being taken into that light by friends and relatives who have already passed over. When a person passes into spirit, they are said to experience great joy and peace, but this can be marred by the realisation that those they have left behind are so distressed. Therefore, however difficult you may find this, try and feel peace and joy for the newly departed soul.

When the person has died, it is usual for them to be either buried or cremated. In the West, cremation is becoming more widespread. Occultly speaking, this fulfils two main purposes: it hastens the release of the soul-enshrouding subtle vehicle from the etheric body, and in the case of a diseased body, the ashes that are then returned to the earth are 'cleansed by fire', thus preventing pollution to the earth.

If we look at how death is dealt with by different cultures, we will see that for most of them death is accepted as part of living and the whole family or community becomes involved in the death process. For the majority of these people, death is not something to be feared but is looked upon as a transformation which allows the person to function at a different vibrational frequency. I feel that studying the way death is handled in these cultures and searching within ourselves for the true meaning of death will help us to overcome the fear that this subject incites. Logically speaking, the only certain thing in life is death.

Some of the ancient customs have been passed down through the ages and can be seen today in some of our modern ceremonies. Unlike our modern society, earlier generations made provision for their loved ones to die at home in familiar surroundings with their friends and family gathered round. Death was an accepted part of life in these communities, not something that happened elsewhere. This is not the case with our present society, in which the act of dying is separated from everyday life. Today the dying are placed in hospitals and hospices away from familiar surroundings, separated from those they love. When death does come it is a cold, clinical event. Shortly afterwards the body is taken to the mortuary and then to the undertakers (where friends and relatives can view the body if they wish), until it is buried or cremated. Is this segregation through the last stage of our life healthy? Does it prolong the grief? I personally believe it does.

APPROACHES TO DEATH

The myths surrounding death and man's loss of immortality are numerous. According to many African people there was originally no death. Its arrival is thought to be due to the transgression either of human beings or of some animal. The Nuer pastoralists of the Southern Sudan tell how there was once a rope joining Heaven and Earth and anyone who grew old climbed the rope and was made young again by the High God before returning to Earth. One day a weaver bird and a hyena are said to have climbed the rope and entered heaven. On seeing them the High God issued instructions that they were to be watched and prevented from returning to Earth, where it was suspected that they would cause trouble. One night they escaped and when they neared the ground the hyena cut the rope, preventing human beings from reaching Heaven. This resulted in them growing old and dying.

Aboriginal myth treats death as the consequence of human misdeeds. Aborigines believe that through spite, foolishness and greed, the gift of immortality slipped beyond the grasp of humankind and was retained only by the moon, which waxes and wanes every month and by the crab, which casts its old battered shell to grow a new one.

According to an Eskimo myth, for a long time there was no such thing as death; people were periodically rejuvenated. This led to the population becoming so large that it threatened to tip up the land and plunge everyone into the sea. Then an old woman, seeing the danger, used magical words to summon death and war. Through this the world was lightened and universal catastrophe averted.

Different cultures have different customs associated with death and dying.

Neanderthal graves have been found to contain remnants of flowers, suggesting that from the earliest times the dead were buried with some form of ceremony. This was confirmed when a Neanderthal skeleton strewn with red ochre and black manganese dioxide was discovered in a grave in France. The black was to obscure the identity of the corpse and red symbolised the renewal of life in the spirit world. Later discoveries of graves belonging to Cro-Magnon man tend to confirm this. Their dead always had red ochre smeared over their body and over the grave and were accompanied by necklaces and joints of meat for their use in the afterworld.

The Tiwi tribes of the Melville and Bathurst islands bury the body of their dead immediately but the funeral ritual is delayed for several months until the grief of family members has subsided. At the funeral, or *pukimani* ceremony, brightly coloured poles are erected to mark the grave, the number of poles varying with the age and status of the deceased. The poles symbolise the link between the worlds of the living and the dead.

Until stopped by missionaries early in the twentieth century, it was the custom of the Worora tribe of the Western Kimberleys in Australia to lay a dead person's body on a burial platform until the flesh had decayed. The remaining bones would then be placed in a cave in the deceased's own territory. If the burial platform was not carefully constructed, the native cats could at times be seen eating the corpse.

For the Alaskan Indians, dying is a very natural and sometimes welcomed process. Members of the tribe know when their death is imminent and will call loved ones to attend their passing. When death occurs, the whole community partakes in the ceremony. They make the coffin, dig the grave, make paper flowers to place on the grave and after the burial service the entire village enjoys a great feast. The Alaskans believe in an afterworld and have many legends about it and about evil spirits, which they believe take the form of animals such as the wolverines. After the death of one of their tribe, these evil spirits are bribed to stop them harming the living or haunting the community.

The Chinese culture believes that the only certainty in life is death. They believe that both good and evil spirits hover around the dead and for this reason it is customary for a patient to die in hospital in preference to their home to prevent evil spirits entering and haunting the home. When a funeral takes place there is much wailing and weeping and if there are only a few members of the deceased's family in attendance, professional mourners are hired to make sure the soul has a good 'send off'. Paper money is burnt in the belief that it will be used by the deceased in the afterworld.

The Japanese proclaim that death should not be feared. They believe that the soul of the deceased is transported after death to a place of great beauty. In order to assure the soul's safe arrival in the afterworld, certain religious practices are observed. These include *yakan*, the bathing of the dead, followed by a bedside service. This service gives the officiating priest an opportunity to console the bereaved.

Of the world's great religions, Hinduism has no founder but has a book of texts known as the *Veda*, a word meaning 'wisdom' or 'knowledge'. The *Veda* proclaims the doctrine of reincarnation, reasoning that a soul must keep returning to mortal existence until it has learned all the lessons necessary to attain enlightenment. It teaches that the soul of the deceased reincarnates immediately after death and if the person has lived a good life their soul will incarnate into another human form but if their life has been selfish and corrupt they incarnate into an animal form.

When death occurs the body is purified by washing the feet with milk and by placing a small amount of water into the mouth. The final act of purification is burning the body by fire, which takes place at the earliest opportunity. To set the pyre ablaze, only pure ghee is used; any other substance is thought to invoke evil spirits.

Islam, founded by the prophet Mohammed in the seventh century at Mecca in Arabia, has its beliefs set down in the Koran. Moslems believe that after the body of the deceased has been buried, two angels appear to question it on its belief in Islam. If the questions are answered correctly, a door opens to allow the soul entry into paradise but if wrong answers are given, a door to hell opens, releasing heat and an odious wind. In the 'Tradition', a book used alongside the Koran, there is mention of a bridge over hell which is said to be sharper than a sword and finer than a hair. All must attempt to cross it. Believers arrive safely but unbelievers fall into the abyss.

Judaism places great sanctity on life and its preservation. With this comes the dilemma on how long life should be preserved and when should a person be allowed to die naturally. The Jewish tradition views the period of terminal illness and dying as a time when loved ones should surround and comfort the patient. Prior to death the patient is encouraged to make their confession, as this is viewed as an important element in the transition of the soul to the afterworld. The deathbed confessional is regarded as a means of reconciliation with God and is structured to be comforting rather than distressing. When death does occur, unless it is of absolute necessity, no autopsy is permitted and the body is buried within 48 hours.

In the Catholic tradition of Ireland, wherever possible a person dies in their own home. Just prior to death they are encouraged to make their confession and are then given the last rites of the church. This ensures that at the Day of Judgement, they will be taken up into heaven, where they will live for eternity. When death occurs, the body is laid out, usually in the individual's own bed, where friends and families visit to say their farewells. This is known as 'the wake', a tradition which allows for the expression of grief and sorrow. The funeral normally takes place within three days of the death and on the set day the undertaker and priest arrive at the house of the deceased. The body is put into the coffin and the priest and mourners walk to the church for the burial service. The Catholic religion teaches that the body will rise again at the final Day of Judgement. For this reason, cremation is not accepted by the faithful.

When I was visiting Ireland, the next-door neighbour to the person I was staying with died. From the time of his death to his funeral, a constant stream of visitors called. These included Irish children who are brought up to accept death as a natural occurrence and not shielded from it. I found this attitude towards death very healthy.

BEYOND DEATH

Some branches of the Christian Church teach that a person who has lived a sinful life will burn in the fires of hell, while others teach that sinners spend their time in purgatory. I personally do not believe such places exist. It has been reported by those who have had near-death experiences that after leaving their physical body they travel down a tunnel at the end of which is a very bright light. At a certain stage of this journey they report seeing the whole of their life being enacted before their eyes. They say that they are made to feel the pain they have caused others and witness their missed opportunities. If they were addicted to drugs, nicotine or alcohol, the craving for these substances remains when they pass over but there are no means for satisfying them. I believe that the hell talked about by the Church is the clearing of these addictive substances from the astral body and the regret and pain felt when our life is passed before us. But after witnessing and learning from the mistakes of the life just finished, the soul moves forward to experience the love and beauty of the spirit world and to take advantage of the many schools of learning found there.

The stages of death have been outlined by Theosophists and other esoteric religions. These stem from the teachings of two Theosophists, H. P. Blavatsky and Alice Bailey. They taught that just prior to death, the soul 'rings out its sound' to broadcast that it has started the withdrawal process from the physical body. This sound sends vibrations along the nadis in the etheric body to release it from its tie to the nervous system and the physical body. The endocrine glands, in response to this sound, release a substance into the bloodstream which affects the heart and causes loss of consciousness. The connection between the nadis and the nervous system is then broken to free the etheric body. The etheric and other subtle bodies constituting the aura then start to withdraw from the physical body. This can be from either one of the two primary or the intermediary exit points. The two primary exits are the top of the head, thought to be used by those who were intellectuals and/or spiritually orientated during their earthly life, and the solar plexus, used by those who displayed in their life strong emotional traits or had little or no spiritual orientation. The intermediary exit, lying just below the apex of the heart, is used by kind and well-meaning individuals.

The subtle bodies emerge from the physical in gradual stages at the chosen point of exit. Although freed from the physical body, the etheric sheath is still magnetically attracted and this is the reason why clairvoyants claim to see the spiritual being standing close by the body. The final stage in this dying process is for the soul to shake itself free from the etheric, which must then die with the physical body.

What is important to remember is the support that is given to the individual passing through these stages of death by their loved ones already in spirit and by the order of angelic beings whose job it is to assist this process. When I have attended the dying, I have experienced the dying person looking at a particular spot in the room and uttering the name of a loved one who has already passed over. I have also seen the joy of recognition that lights a face just prior to death, but what has never failed to fill me with awe is the emptiness of the physical form when the soul has departed.

When the soul has left the physical body, it goes to the plane of existence to which it is most suited. The master Christ said: 'In my Father's house are many mansions.' I believe that he was referring to these different levels of afterlife existence. Peter Richelieu in his book *A Soul's Journey* (Aquarian Press, 1958) names these levels of existence as the astral, mental and causal planes and suggests that each plane has within it seven different levels. This knowledge comes from the experiences he had after the death of his brother. While sitting and mourning his loss, he was greeted by a spirit being who over many nights taught him how to consciously leave his body while it slept. While out of his body, the spirit master took him to several of the spiritual planes to experience life there. In his book Richelieu describes the beauty of these places and some of the beings he encountered. These included devas (the guardians of the plant kingdom), angelic beings and the souls of those already departed. He talks about the schools of learning that exist in the spirit worlds and the evolution of the animal kingdom.

A HARMONIOUS DEATH

If we are able to accept that we are spiritual beings living in a human body and when the time comes for us to leave the Earth plane we return to our natural spiritual home, then death will become for us a very natural occurrence that holds no fear. As Michael Eastcott in *The Phenomenon of Death* (Sundial House, 1976) writes 'Death, if we could but realise it, is one of our most practised activities. Death is essentially a matter of consciousness.' He explains that we are conscious one moment on the physical plane, and the next moment we have withdrawn on to another plane and are actively conscious there. As long as we identify consciousness with being on the physical plane, death will remain something to be feared. But as soon as we accept that we also exist as souls and that we can focus our consciousness or sense of awareness in any form or on any plane at will, or 'in any direction within the form of God', then the concept of 'death' will no longer exist.

Eastcott continues by saying that although this is a liberating process for a dying individual, death still presents problems. The first is the grief and sorrow of relatives and friends that are left behind. Their emotional upset and attempts to cling on to the dying person can hinder the smooth departure of the spiritual being from the physical body. The second is the bewilderment of the dying one faced by the 'dead' person when they find themselves in the unfamiliar conditions of non-physical life. Both of these problems will be resolved once humanity realises that the non-physical condition after death is not new at all, but really very old. We have all 'died' many times before and will most probably do so again many times in the future.

It has been said that fear is the outstanding attitude associated with death. We can attribute this largely to inadequate education. Just as intense effort during recent decades has assisted in making gentle and conscious childbirth available to Western women, so the efforts of many health professionals and psychologists are helping remove the taboo from death. Eliminating the fear of death is a vital task of our time.

The following information is taken from Master Djwal Kul's, (known as DK), comments on overcoming the fear of death: DK is known as one of the ascended masters. As a young man he left his home to study with a Secret Society of advanced initiates in a secluded lamasery in the Tibetan Himalayas. DK explains that our fear of death is due to the emphasis which we put upon the physical body and how we identify ourselves with it; it is based also upon an innate fear of loneliness and the loss of the familiar. But the sense of isolation experienced after death, when the man finds himself without a physical vehicle, is nothing compared to the loneliness at birth. When we are born the soul finds itself immersed in a body which, at first, it cannot take care of itself and through which it cannot establish intelligent contact with surrounding conditions for a long period of time. The new soul does not recall the identities or significance of the group of souls with which he finds himself in relationship. This loneliness disappears only gradually as he makes his own contacts and gathers around him those whom he calls his friends.

After death on the other plane of existence we find ourselves amongst those who have been connected with us in our physical life. We are also aware of those still in physical bodies; we can see them, and tune into their emotions and their thinking.

If we are to have death that is free from fear, we need to make preparations for it during our life. If as practitioners we choose to work with the dying we need to have eliminated all fear of death in ourselves. As healers, let us carry the torch that will light the way for others as they approach this stage in their life. Let us develop an attitude of living that embraces both sides of the portal we call 'death'. Let us rejoice in our physical bodies, but let us not lose sight of our true, non-physical being – the soul. Let us learn to listen to the soul and respond joyously to its call, whether this call be for birth, for death or for life beyond both these events.

POSTSCRIPT

THE MAITREYA SCHOOL gave its students a list of 'seed thoughts' to provide food for reflection in relation to the question: 'What are the qualities of a colour practitioner?' I use these with my own students and would like to share them with you. The best way of working with them is to take each one separately and meditate upon it for two to three days to listen to what it is saying to you.

- The healer recognises life as a flowing process and supports the patient within the movement of their individual process.
- The healer radiates healing energy by the potency and purity of their 'Beingness'. Being healing overshadows doing healing.
- The healer seeks to serve – neither as a submissive slave nor as a directive authority but as a source of strength and as a beam of light which helps others find their way to wholeness.
- The healer strives to reveal and nurture wholeness in themselves, in the patient and in the world.
- The healer accepts responsibility – the ability to respond. This ability to respond depends upon cultivating the qualities of compassion, purity of motive, insightful understanding, selflessness, good will, self-mastery and 'the silence that sounds'.
- The healer recognises their work as a way of life and strives to be a healing presence at all times, in all places and under all conditions.
- The healer celebrates life and fears neither birth nor death nor any changes in form.

- The healer works from a point of joy.
- The healer brings light, shares love and offers the power of choice.

Lily Cornford always taught that all future ideas will carry us to a fuller, holistic, more co-operative, more energetic array of healing techniques that will lead to the recognition that true healing eventuates when the life of the soul can flow through our personality without encountering any impediments, hindrances, congestion or obstruction. This will require a new outlook on healing and healers. Instead of focusing on health and disease, prevention and wellness will be encouraged, with the realisation that health is only the tip of the iceberg, a tip supported by the submerged, unnoticed areas of lifestyle, behaviour, psychological habits and philosophical understanding of our place in the universe.

When this happens we will become transformers rather than healers. No longer will we be limited to patching up and cleaning up damaged bodies. We will know the spiritual essence of every human being and we will be adept at nurturing, stimulating and supporting each individual in the process of releasing and realising that essence, thereby allowing each individual to discover the power of self-healing and self-transformation on Earth and prepare the way through unconditioned love for a fuller, more creative and more loving humanity, a humanity willing to serve rather than be served, to love rather than be loved, sharing universal light rather than seeking that light.

For all this, healing – the return to wholeness, the restoration of balance, the 'lifting of the downward focused eyes unto the healer within the form' – is only the beginning. All of this is only the beginning. The learning and growing never stop.

PROFESSIONAL TRAINING AND TREATMENT

A T THE TIME OF writing this book a great deal is happening in the complementary medical field to improve training standards. This will ensure that those qualifying will have reached a high standard of professionalism in both the theory and practice of their chosen therapy. This is an excellent step forward and one which will help to eliminate those people who take one or two weekend courses and then proceed to set themselves up as practitioners. All that these people do is give complementary therapy a bad name through their lack of knowledge and experience. There is no member of the public who would knowingly allow themselves to be treated by a medical doctor with inadequate training, therefore why should complementary therapists be allowed to do this? If we hope to share an equal footing with allopathic medicine and be accepted by the medical profession, we need to be able to show them that our level of training and professionalism is equal to theirs and I am happy to report that there are great moves afoot to achieve this.

THE COLOUR PRACTITIONER DIPLOMA

At present the colour practitioner diploma course takes a minimum of two years and some of the topics covered are the physics of light, the history of colour therapy, the subtle anatomy, the vibrational energies of visible light, their administration and use, the metaphysical cause of disease, first aid and counselling, which plays a major role. Each student is expected to do approximately 60 hours of practical work alongside essays and a dissertation on any aspect of colour they care to research. During their first year they must study anatomy and physiology and the second year pathology and disease. Another important aspect of the colour practitioner diploma course is personal growth, because a student needs to work through their own problems before trying to help others work with theirs. As many of the great masters have said: 'Physician, heal thyself before trying to help others to do the same.'

Some colour schools embody a second complementary discipline into their syllabus. One frequently incorporated is sound. Colour and sound have a very close affinity to each other and work well together. Another is sacred geometry. The two-dimensional shapes of the platonic solids amplify the power of colour when used with it. These shapes are found in our own cellular structure and some types of viruses have been found to reflect them.

When planning to take a colour practitioner diploma course, it is advisable to request the syllabus from several schools to find the one most suited to your needs. After making your choice, it is recommended that you write to the Complementary Medical Association (CMA) enclosing a stamped addressed envelope, to find out if the school you have selected is teaching to the required standard and therefore approved by them. Alternatively, you may wish to contact them first to find the names of recommended schools and then write to these for information. The same applies if you are looking for a colour practitioner. The CMA will be able to give you the name of a qualified practitioner in your area or direct you to a colour school for the name of a practitioner qualified through them.

OTHER COURSES

Apart from running training courses, there are a number of schools who run introductory days on the vibrational energies of colour. These are designed for those who wish to know more about the subject before embarking upon a long training course. I would recommend these. There are also courses available which teach the integration of colour with another complementary therapy. The Oracle School of Colour runs a certificated course on the integration of colour with reflexology. To be eligible to enrol for this a student must hold a reflexology qualification from a recognised school. The level to which colour is taught on this course qualifies a reflexologist to use colour only on the reflexes of the hands and feet.

CORRESPONDENCE COURSES

There are at present a number of colour therapy correspondence courses and I personally feel that these leave a lot to be desired. Their main drawback is the lack of personal contact with other students, lack of practical experience and the lack of opportunity for personal growth. The techniques taught for applying colour are varied and sometimes complex and these cannot be learnt just by reading about them. I am sure that there is nobody who would be happy to be registered with a doctor who had done most if not all his training through a correspondence course. Expertise is gained through practice, which allows for mistakes to be made and rectified. During the many courses that I have run, I have seen students grow and blossom as they worked with each other and with themselves. Most student groups become a safe integrated unit where it is permissible to break down and cry and where friendship, trust, understanding and love is given as emotional and mental clutter accumulated over many years is worked through and released.

STARTING OUT

Once a person has qualified they usually choose to work either at a complementary clinic or set up their own practice. Sometimes it is possible for them to work for a short time at the school where they were trained. From my own experience at being allowed to work with Lily for a year, I would recommend this. If this is not an option, I would suggest that you work for a time in a clinic with other complementary therapists. This will help you to gain confidence as well as having other practitioners to talk to. Another benefit is not having the immediate expense of equipping your own therapy room.

Some therapists find it advantageous to put aside a percentage of their earnings each week towards buying their equipment when they start their own practice. When the time for this venture comes you will need to find either in the vicinity of your home or in your home a room to use for this purpose. If the room is in your home, it should be kept only for the purpose of treating. The room should be pleasantly decorated, kept spotlessly clean and only have in it the things needed for your work.

If you are orientated towards playing soft background music during a treatment session, it is advisable to ask the patient if they would welcome this and what type of music helps them to relax. What we find peaceful and soothing may do disastrous things to someone else. If I decide to use music for a particular patient I usually ask them to bring a tape of the music they would like played. I remember running a yoga class for teenagers and at the end of each session I would take them into relaxation and then play music while they relaxed. The only music they found helpful was pop. It did wonders for them but left me exhausted.

When starting your own practice you will initially have to advertise but after some time your practice should grow through recommendation. A question I am frequently asked by students is the length of time it takes to establish a practice. The answer is dependent upon how good you are as a practitioner. Another question which arises is the treatment fee. Again, this will be governed by the location of your practice, your overheads and the time spent treating. It is usual for fees to be higher in large cities than in rural districts.

One golden rule for all practitioners to observe is patient confidentiality. Anything discussed or any information imparted by the patient should never be disclosed to another person without the patient's permission. If you feel you need to discuss any of your patients with another practitioner, their permission should first be sought. I frequently reassure my patients by telling them that anything discussed during a therapy session is never repeated. After qualifying a student is given a code of ethics by the school and this they are expected to abide by.

Once you have qualified and before you start treating patients you need to have insurance cover. If you work from your home this should include personal liability to cover you should a patient fall down the stairs or trip over and hurt themselves. Some insurance companies have a multi-insurance pack and this includes things like damage to equipment and loss of income to yourself through sickness or an accident. Most schools will provide the names of insurance companies that deal with complementary therapy but sometimes it is advisable to shop around for a better deal.

Of equal importance is keeping a record of all treatment carried out for a patient. In the unlikely event of something going wrong and the patient taking legal action, you may need to produce these records as evidence. There have been occasions when a patient attends for treatment after being abused or ill treated by another practitioner. If the patient decides to sue the first practitioner you may be asked to give evidence. If you have failed to keep accurate records, this will be almost impossible to do and, in law, may go against you.

When you start to work as a self-employed person, you will need to keep accounts of your income and expenditure for tax purposes. Under expenditure you can include expenses incurred for equipment, white coats, couch roll, etc. If working from your home you may be able to include part of your telephone bill and the heating for the room you are using. The best person to advise you about all of this would be an accountant. After initially seeking advice, a lot of practitioners then continue with self-assessment.

Gaining a diploma in complementary therapy shows that you have acquired the basic skills to practise, you have laid your foundation. Having done so, the next step is to start building on this by researching colour and exploring the ways other practitioners are working with it.

What I feel is important to remember is the fact that no new discoveries or insights are exclusively ours. We have just been privileged in having these communicated to us by that universal light for the benefit of our patients and for others working in the field of colour. Therefore for the good of the whole field of colour, we need to share these ideas with our colleagues and not keep them exclusively for ourselves, claiming them as our own because they are not. All this knowledge is a mere rediscovery of what has gone before.

RECOMMENDED READING

The Angel Oracle, Ambika Wauters, Connections (1996)

The Beginner's Guide to Colour Psychology, Angela Wright, Kyle Cathie Ltd (1995)

The Bodymind Workbook, Debbie Shapiro, Element (1990)

The Chakras, Naomi Ozaniec, Element (1990)

Colour Healing, Lilian Verner Bonds, Lorenz Books (1999)

Colour Healing, Mary Anderson, The Aquarian Press (1979)

Colour Healing, Pauline Wills, Piatkus (1998)

Colour Me Healing: Colourpuncture: A New Medicine of Light, Jack Allanach, Element (1997)

Colour Psychology And Colour Therapy, Faber Birren, Citadel Press (1950)

Colour Therapy, Dr Reuben Amber, Aurora Press (1983)

Colour Therapy, Pauline Wills, Element Books (1993)

Colour Your Life, Howard & Dorothy Sun, Piatkus (1998)

Discover the Magic of Colour, Lilian Verner Bonds, Optima (1993)

The Eighth Key to Colour, Ronald Hunt, L.N. Fowler & Co. Ltd (1965)

Healing with Colour, Helen Graham, Gill & Macmillan (1996)

The Healing Power of Colour Zone Therapy, Joseph Corvo & Lilian Verner-Bonds, Piatkus (1998)

The Healer's Hand Book, Georgina Regan & Debbie Shapiro, Element (1988)

In Search of Schrödinger's Cat, John Gribbin, Black Swan (1991)

Intermediate Studies of the Human Aura, Djwal Kul, Summit University Press (1974)

Light Years Ahead – The illustrated guide to Full Spectrum and Colored Light in Mindbody Healing, Light Years Ahead Production (1996)

Man's Subtle Bodies and Centres, Omraam Mikhaël Aïvanhov, Prosveta (1986)

On Death and Dying, Elisabeth Kübler-Ross, Routledge (1970)

On Life After Death, Elisabeth Kübler-Ross, Celestial Arts (1991)

Reflexology and Colour Therapy, Pauline Wills, Element (1992)

The Reflexology Handbook, Laura Norman, Piatkus (1998)

Relativity & Quantum Physics, Roger Muncaster, Stanley Thornes Ltd (1995)

Spiritual Aspects of the Healing Arts, Dora Kunz (ed.), The Theosophical Publishing House (1985)

The Symbolism of Colour, Ellen Conroy, Newcastle Publishing Co. (1966)
The Symbolism of Colour, Faber Birren, Citadel Press (1988)
Teach Yourself to Meditate, Eric Harrison, Piatkus (1997)
Theory of Colours, Johann Wolfgang von Goethe, MIT Press (1970)
Vibrational Medicine, Richard Gerber, Bear & Co. (1988)
Working with Colour: a beginner's guide, Pauline Wills, Headway (1977)
Working With Your Chakras, Ruth White, Piatkus (1997)
Your Healing Power, Jack Angelo, Piatkus (1998)

INDEX